ACUPUNCTURE ENERGETICS

ACUPUNCTURE ENERGETICS

A Workbook for Diagnostics and Treatment

Mark Seem, Ph.D.
Dipl. Ac. (NCCA)

Healing Arts Press
Rochester, Vermont

Healing Arts Press
One Park Street
Rochester, Vermont 05767
www.InnerTraditions.com

Healing Arts Press is a division of Inner Traditions International

Note to the reader: This book is intended as an informational guide. The remedies, approaches, and techniques described herein are meant to supplement, and not to be a substitute for, professional medical care or treatment. They should not be used to treat a serious ailment without prior consultation with a qualified health care professional.

LIBRARY OF CONGRESS CATALOGING-IN-PUBLICATION DATA
Seem, Mark
    Acupuncture energetics : a workbook for diagnostics and treatment
/ Mark Seem.
        p.   cm.
    Reprint. Originally published: Wellinborough, Northamptonshire ;
Rochester, Vt. : Thorson's Pub. Group, 1987.
    Includes bibliographical references and index.
    ISBN 0-89281-435-7
    1. Acupuncture.   I. Title.
RM184.S36   1991
615.8'92--dc20   91-2861
                                                            CIP

Printed and bound in the United States.

10 9 8 7 6 5

Note

TABLE OF CONTENTS

ACKNOWLEDGEMENTS

This workbook is indebted to Bryan Manuele, Dipl. Ac. (NCCA), with whom I thought through many of the concepts contained herein, and to the students at the Midwest Center for the Study of Oriental Medicine, the Tri-State Institute of Traditional Chinese Acupuncture and the Traditional Acupuncture Institute who allowed me to try these notions out with them.

Finally, this workbook owes special thanks to Elaine Stern, Dipl. Ac. (NCCA) who typed the manuscript and edited the case histories.

PREFACE: How to Use this Book

This workbook is intended for students in their second or third year, and practitioners and teachers of acupuncture. It is structured in such a way that the reader moves from a theoretical discussion of energetic diagnostics in Traditional Chinese Medicine, to the development of a problem-solving approach to diagnosis. The second half of the workbook consists of a review of Zang–Fu syndromes with exercises that will afford the reader a far stronger grasp of these syndromes. Finally, there are dozens of cases to be worked through to internalize the problem-solving approach to diagnosis contained in the first part of the text.

Wherever possible we have keyed cases to two main texts, *The Essentials of Chinese Acupuncture*, and *The Web That Has No Weaver: Understanding Chinese Medicine*. In this way, someone who carefully works through all the exercises in the book and who checks their responses against the pages indicated for the above texts, will have internalized the major Zang–Fu syndromes of Traditional Chinese Medicine and gained increased familiarity and a working knowledge of the main texts in the field.

Finally, teachers should work through the text as well, and use it to reinforce their classroom teaching. An answer key to all cases appears in the Appendix.

INTRODUCTION

The Eight Principal Patterns serve . . . as a conceptual matrix
that enables the physician to organize the relationship between
particular clinical signs and Yin and Yang.[1]

The diagnosis Chinese Medicine strives for and produces is,
by definition, a synthesis of numerous individual factors,
*assembled in each patient examined in a unique and
characteristic manner* [my italics][2]

Acupuncture energetic diagnosis begins, always, with the
patient's *presence* and *present*, and is finely attuned to data of
energetic significance. While the practitioner of Chinese
medicine, and here we are referring to the West, must pay
attention to everything that the patient has to say, as well as
his movements, temperament, structure, etc., he must be
especially attentive, on a deeper level, to information that
helps him begin to approach the nature of what Kaptchuk
terms the 'pattern of disharmony' that the patient presents
with. The determination as to what information among the
myriad signs and symptoms is of importance is guided by the
practitioner's keen awareness of energetics. Energetics is the
essence of the Chinese medical system, and consists of the
various regular and secondary meridian systems (the internal
and external pathways), the Zang and Fu (viscera seen
functionally, energetically), the various forms of Qi
(specifically Wei, Ying and Jing), Blood, Body Fluids and
Shen (emotional, spiritual factors). Energetics is not
anthropomorphic, and evaluations of energetic disturbances
do not remain at the manifest level, but seek to clarify a more
essential but less visible reality. As in particle physics, the
problem is one of inferring, on the basis of the energetic

traces left behind by the movements of particles through a force field, information about the nature of the particular particles and their configurations. While one cannot always see the actual movement of energy in such a context, one can begin to assess its effects. Chinese diagnosis is aimed at evaluating energetic effects within the force field of the patient's body, and begins with the distressing signals present in the here-and-now, the patient's *present* — in order to attempt to solve the problem of where the present disturbance emanates from (the *past*), and in order to make certain predictions about where it might evolve to (the *future*).

Psychoanalysis, another energetic science, was defined by Freud as a *depth* psychology. What he meant by this was that the analyst had to learn how to see through and underneath the patient's verbiage, avoiding much camouflaging along the way, in order to perceive the primary process of the unconscious functionings. A good analyst may well seem very remote, even distant, perceived from the outside, but he and the patient know full well that the process they are engaged in has little to do with the conventions of social discourse, and is aimed at enabling the patient to learn something from a more hidden space in his body about his own functioning in the world, his particular symptoms, his diseases and defences. The task of the analyst, seen in this light, consists in learning to perceive those clues enunciated by the patient that enable the patient to see his inner functionings more clearly. A psychoanalyst is a detective whose mystery is the patient's soul.

Chinese medicine functions in a way not unlike psychoanalysis. It is a depth science. It does not stay at the level of what the patient wishes to speak about, but is attentive to energetic clues that lead to perceiving patterns of disharmony within the patient's body, seen as a force field. A good practitioner must listen and see differently in order to understand the energetic nature of the disturbance, and thereby initiate an energetic treatment. While probably not practised in the East, a Western practitioner of Chinese medicine would do well to educate the patient about his or her patterns of energetic distress and dysfunction. This, in turn, will enable the patient to understand his/her own signals of disharmony and take responsibility for doing something about it.

In brief then, the practitioner of Chinese medical diagnosis knows how to listen for energetic data and knows which information to key in on. Energetics begins with the patient's signs and symptoms and seeks to perceive a pattern within them. The tone of the patient's voice, the way he carries himself, his colour or emotions, will be no less important data in this regard than the colour of the patient's tongue fur and urine, the fact that there are loose stools containing undigested food particles or that there are pains that migrate about. The practitioner must not privilege certain, more objective data, over other, more subjective data, but rather weave together these pieces of information to construct a plausible energetic 'story'. All symptoms, all signs, all emissions from the patient's body are an integral part of a language of energetics that enables the practitioner to assess the current state of the patient's forces.

At this point we would like to turn to a discussion of Chinese Energetic Diagnosis, and present one way of breaking it down for the Western practitioner. While our problem-solving approach may not strike the reader as purely Chinese, we wish to stress that Western practitioners of Oriental Medicine must discover ways of making Chinese diagnosis work for them, while keeping intimately in touch with the essence of this diagnostic system, namely energetics. No major books on Chinese medicine written in English explain how one goes from gathering information (the Four Examinations) to ordering a treatment. Many steps are missing, at least for us. Westerners cannot learn Chinese medicine like the Chinese learn it (memorization). Our education is different, our way of learning is different, and we must be innovative. In this regard, books such as those by Kaptchuk, Van Nghi or Porkert are often of far greater use to us than translations of Chinese texts. This is because these Western authors have had to grapple with Chinese medicine in terms of presenting it to a Western readership. Hopefully the days of blind adherence to the Chinese texts will give way to creative thinking of our own: the American acupuncturist will then develop his own literature, and make important additions and advances in the field.

1.

YIN-YANG AND THE FIVE PHASES

The false distinction between 'Eight-Principle acupuncture' and 'Five-Element' acupuncture, while indeed false, is a reality in American acupuncture today. Essentially the issue arose because American practitioners reacted in one of two major ways to acupuncture and Traditional Chinese Medicine as evolved in the People's Republic of China during and after the Cultural Revolution. Many, although familiar with Five Elements in the work of Mary Austin and Lawson and Wood, felt attracted to *An Outline of Chinese Acupuncture* because it came directly from the People's Republic, and thus had to be closer to 'true' acupuncture. This caused those more strongly grounded in Five Elements to conclude that these other practitioners, and this other acupuncture, were symptomatic and a perversion of the true science and art of traditional Chinese acupuncture. When *The Essentials of Chinese Acupuncture* appeared, many in the pro-China camp reacted with joy to this reformulation of *The Outline*, as it contained valuable information on diagnosis, and especially on the 'Eight Principles' that clarified much for those working from what has now become known as the TCM model. The fact that a few states chose *The Essentials* as the major text from which to draw their tests did nothing to alleviate this dilemma. What became clear, however, once practitioners, and essentially educators from both 'camps' came together during the meetings that led to the development of the National Council of Acupuncture Schools and Colleges, was that the demons both groups imagined to exist were to a great extent phantoms with no real existence. As we all began to teach and learn from each other it became ever more clear that the real issue was not one's stance on

TCM or Traditional Acupuncture, but rather the need to clearly begin to formulate what American acupuncture is, and what we wanted it to be. In so doing, it is crucial that we learn the Chinese concepts and methods carefully, before choosing sides. Again, the works of Porkert, Kaptchuk and Van Nghi serve us well here.

The reason that we stated that the distinction between Five Elements and Eight Principles is a false one is because the real issue is concerned with 'Five Elements *and* Yin and Yang'. All of Chinese medical philosophy derives from the notions of Yin and Yang, including the Five Elements or Phases, and the Eight Guiding criteria (to use Porkert's term) are simply an extension of Yin and Yang. One cannot do Chinese energetic diagnosis without utilizing both Yin and Yang and the Five Phases, as we shall attempt to demonstrate.[3]

The Five Phases constitute an abstract system that enables the practitioner to locate which element or phase is affected and to make certain deductions about the possible *past* (C.F., or Causative Factor, as it is termed by some) of the disorder, as well as possible *futures* (that it will go from Wood to Fire along the generation cycle, or to Earth along the destruction cycle, etc.). But it is not sufficient to help one determine whether the disorder is on the surface or deep, and it does not help one state much about the nature of the disturbance within the element itself. The Five Phases and their correspondances (Wood corresponds to Wind, Green, Anger, Nails, Muscles and Tendons, Liver and Gall-bladder. Decision-making, etc.) helps us see that a specific problem exists, say, in Earth, but it doesn't take us very far in defining the nature of this Earth disharmony. This is where Yin and Yang and the Eight Guiding Criteria enable us to systematically categorize every sign and symptom and say much more about the state of the particular phase's imbalance. We have learned from Five Phases that it is in Earth, to continue our example a moment longer, and an Eight Guiding Criteria assessment now tells us that it is in the Yin of Earth (Spleen), in its Yang functions (transportation and transformation), that it is a deficiency of this Yang function, that the nature of the disorder is cold due to this deficiency or Yang (heat) and that this explains the presence of oedema and diarrhoea with loose stools containing undigested food particles. Five Phases helped us determine that the problem was in 'Earth'. The Eight Guiding Criteria enabled us to add that it is a deficiency of Yang of the Spleen. This is a common pattern, borne out daily in the clinic, and there is no way that a Five Phases approach divorced from an evaluation by means of the Eight Guiding Criteria could have arrived at such a detailed diagnosis. On the other hand, a diagnosis arrived at from an Eight Criteria approach, divorced from a knowledge and assessment of the Five Phases would also be insufficient. In brief, the Five Phases keep us focused on the energetic movements of disharmonies which are ever fleeting and the essence of what we are after, while the Eight Guiding Criteria enable us to apply a systematic analysis of all data gathered in a consistent way, in order to

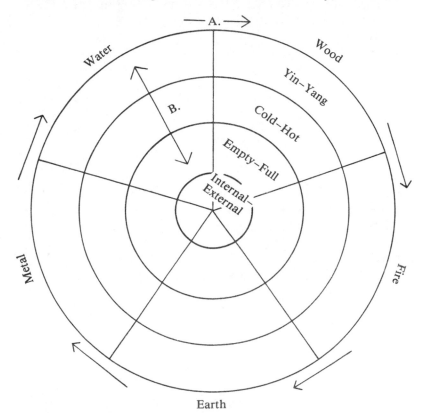

A. The Five changing Movements or Phases.
B. The four constant binary dimensions.

(reprinted from *Journal of Traditional Acupuncture*, Vol 2, 82) measure the patient's pattern of disharmony against the major patterns of Chinese medical pathology. This can be demonstrated in a diagram, where the Five Phases are energetic movements with definite cycles, while the Eight Criteria are the constants that must be assessed in whatever Phase we are investigating.

2.

THE STEPS OF DIAGNOSIS AND TREATMENT PLANNING

One looks at any presenting pattern of disharmony in a patient from several perspectives, each of which represents another outlook that enables us to continuously refine our energetic evaluation. The major perspectives from which we analyse clinical data are clearly Yin–Yang (Eight Guiding Criteria) and the Five Phases or Elements. But we also look at this data that the patient presents us with from the vantage point of the Twelve 'Officials', the Zang and Fu Patterns of Disharmony, the symptomatology of disturbances of the regular and secondary meridian systems, and the patterns of disturbances in Qi, Blood and Body Fluids. The data is assessed from each outlook, in a filtering process that refines one's understanding of the disharmony and enables us to describe its configuration or pattern. The more one knows about the Elements and Officials, the disharmonies of the Zang/Fu, the imbalances of the various meridian systems, and disorders of Qi, Blood and Fluids, the more one's energetic diagnosis will be sophisticated and the closer one will be able to come to the reality of the patient's clinical distress. All of these various pieces of data are helpful and inform the process of energetic diagnosis.[4] They are abstractions useful in guiding the practitioner along the way of diagnosis, and if seen as such will never present the danger of robbing the practitioner of his/her integrity, personal style, approach, ethical considerations and mission. The better informed the practitioner, the more effective his or her treatments will be.

We would like to propose a nine-step process of performing energetic diagnosis that is influenced by a problem-solving approach. Faced with an energetic problem, the practitioner functions much like a detective as he hunts for relevant clues and discards other information that is less important. This hunt consists of several discreet processes which I arbitrarily break up into these nine steps, for educational purposes only. Obviously the good practitioner no longer thinks linearly, from step 1 to 9. But for didactic purposes, students would do well to begin this way, in order to develop good diagnostic habits. The nine steps are as follows.

1. *Differentiation of each sign and symptom*: Here one lists the various signs and symptoms as they occur and states as much as one can about each (example: yellow tongue coating = heat): It is important, for didactic reasons, not to try to reach a diagnosis at this point. Just state what each sign or symptom might mean by free association from whatever perspectives you utilize.

2. *Determination of the presence or absence of exogenous pathogenic factors* (pernicious influences or perverse energies): State whether these factors play a role in the presenting disturbance, and name the pernicious influences involved (example: Cold and Wind).

3. *Determination of whether the disturbance is of the Zang/Fu or the meridians* (example: a disturbance of the Liver in its spreading functions, as opposed to the tendino-muscular meridian of the Liver, whose symptoms might look decidedly similar).

4. *Evaluation of all clinical data in terms of the Eight Guiding Criteria*: State whether the disorder is internal or external, deficient or excess, cold or hot (if appropriate) and Yin or Yang.

5. *Establishment of a working diagnosis*: One now gathers together all information gleaned from the above procedures and makes a final determination utilizing Eight Guiding Criteria and Five Phases, of a working diagnosis. This diagnosis will possibly be changed or refined in successive treatments, but must be articulated enough to lead to a treatment plan. No diagnosis is final in an energetic science.

6. *Determination of the treatment principle*: Based on the working diagnosis, one must ascertain an appropriate treatment principle that delineates whether and how one will treat the acute symptoms ('branches') as opposed to

the underlying energetic imbalance ('roots'). Most often both will be treated simultaneously, but emphasis is usually placed on one or the other. Note that in acute conditions, one almost always tends to the 'branches' first, and only once these are controlled satisfactorily does one proceed with a more etiological treatment.

7. *Choice of treatment strategies*: For example, if the treatment principle was to 'clear the surface' and 'disperse the pernicious influences' the strategy might be to utilize local and distal points according to the treatment of tendino-muscular meridians.

8. *Selection of the methods of treatment*: A decision is made here as to whether to use moxibustion, needling, cupping, herbs, etc.

9. *Selection of appropriate points*: Points are selected based on their energetic functions and appropriateness with respect to the treatment strategy. For example, if we are clearing the surface in a tendino-muscular disorder of the Small Intestine meridian, in addition to draining the local points of the Small Intestine tendino-muscular meridian, one will choose appropriate distal points. While T.H. 5 or L.I. 4 might well be chosen for their energetic effects on the affected region(s), S.I. 3 is more appropriate for a few reasons. Firstly it is on the same path as the disturbance. Secondly, if one is draining the T.M. meridian, which is a superficial meridian system, one would do well also to tonify the associated principal meridian of the Small Intestine to strengthen it so that the disorder on the surface does not become lodged more deeply.

One might add that the obvious next step, always, after step 9 is to continuously reassess the situation and refine one's diagnosis appropriately.

3.

PATTERNS OF THE ZANG-FU REVIEWED

We will begin our discussion of Zang–Fu syndromes by discussing the Yin and Yang of the Kidneys (Water) since they are the root of life. Wood, Fire, Earth and Metal will follow. In the latter four categories you will be asked to close the book and write down normal and abnormal symptomatology for each Zang and Fu, as well as give treatment strategies and points and rationale for common clinical disorders of each energetic phase. In so doing, you will note that the patterns of disharmony in each of the Zang–Fu spheres can be arrived at by merely looking at what must occur, energetically, if a function of Zang or Fu breaks down. This process will enable you to have an organic understanding of patterns of disharmony, rather than just memorizing syndromes.

A final note is in order. One might say that all disharmonies stem, to a greater or lesser extent, from deficiency of the Yin or Yang Root of Life (Yin or Yang of the Kidneys). A deficiency of Yin (water, fluids, cooling), will lead to increasing Yang (fire, drying up of fluids, heating). Hence in deficient Yin root, we will often encounter such disorders as rising fire of the liver, liver yang ascending, heart fire blazing upwards. In other words, If the Yin root is deficient, one's syndromes will be of an uncontrolled Yang type — becoming hot types of disorder, to speak phenomenologically.

Conversely, if the Yang root is deficient (Yang of the Kidneys) there will be disorders where thermoregulation is deficient and the patient will be chilled, prey to cold disorders and have a slow metabolism. These disorders will be of a decreasing Yang type, presenting with increase of cold and a build-up of fluids (dampness) — becoming cold and becoming damp.

Please note that this is a brief review of Zang–Fu energetics, aimed at refreshing the reader's mind concerning common patterns of disharmony. For a more detailed discussion, see the texts listed in the bibliography. The purpose of this review is to place the Zang–Fu disharmonies within the context of Eight Principles and Five Phases, for a better understanding of acupuncture energetic treatment planning.

Water Patterns (Kidneys and Urinary Bladder)

What do we know about Water? (What are its correspondences?)

What are the energetic functions of the Kidneys?

1. Stores Jing, which rules birth, development, maturation, is the source of life and individual development, gives the person the potential to produce life, holds the underlying material of each organ's existence and is the foundation of the body's Yin and of each organ's Yin and Yang (since Yin produces Yang).
2. Stores the essence which is the inherited part from each of the parents and the acquired essence which is transformed from the pure aspect of food.
3. The nourishing, nurturing, moistening, and supportive aspects of life.
4. The Kidney Jing produces marrow, which in turn produces the spinal cord and bones. The bones manufacture blood and teeth (which are the surplus of bone).
5. Fire of the Kidneys. Life Gate Fire (Ming Men). This is the warming, activating and generating activity of the body.
6. Fire of the Kidneys rules the Water. The Fire is the 'pilot light' which transforms the water into a mist and gives the Kidney its vaporizing power.
7. The Lungs send Water to the Kidneys. The Kidneys separate the water into clear and turbid with the clear being retained in the Kidney and the turbid being turned into urine and passed to the Urinary Bladder.
8. Receives and grasps the Qi – Root of the Qi – enables air to penetrate deeply, completing inhalation.

9. Yang is the active part of reproduction – sexuality.

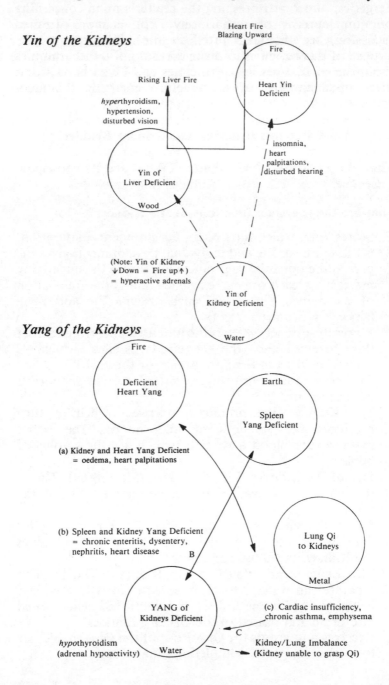

Yin of the Kidneys

Heart Fire
Blazing Upward

Fire

Heart Yin
Deficient

Rising Liver Fire

*hyper*thyroidism,
hypertension,
disturbed vision

insomnia,
heart
palpitations,
disturbed hearing

Yin of
Liver Deficient

Wood

(Note: Yin of Kidney
↓Down = Fire up↑)
= hyperactive adrenals

Yin of
Kidney Deficient

Water

Yang of the Kidneys

Fire

Deficient
Heart Yang

Earth

Spleen
Yang Deficient

(a) Kidney and Heart Yang Deficient
= oedema, heart palpitations

(b) Spleen and Kidney Yang Deficient
= chronic enteritis, dysentery,
nephritis, heart disease   B

Lung Qi
to Kidneys

Metal

YANG of
Kidneys Deficient

(c) Cardiac insufficiency,
chronic asthma, emphysema

C

*hypo*thyroidism   Water
(adrenal hypoactivity)

Kidney/Lung Imbalance
(Kidney unable to grasp Qi)

Kidney Patterns

All Kidney problems are problems of Deficiency. There is no such thing as an Excess problem in the Kidneys. Jing or Essence is a given quantity from birth, and you cannot have too much of it. Yves Requena refers to an Excess of Kidney Yang as a *relative* excess (i.e. if Yin of the Kidney is exhausted, the Yang will be in relative excess).

The Kidney syndromes are rarely isolated syndromes. Since they are the root of all the Yin and Yang organs, a problem with the Kidneys will have a strong effect on the other Zang–Fu.

Deficiency of Yin of the Kidneys may result from a long illness, or from excessive sexual activity. When the Yin fluids are low the body cannot produce marrow for the bones, nor can it nourish the brain, thus producing mental signs mentioned above.

Deficiency of Yang of the Kidneys
Weak Life Gate Fire (deficiency and cold). Bright white or darkish complexion, subdued, quiet manner (no Shen), fear of cold, cold limbs with cold and sore lower back, impotence, sterility, spermatorrhoea, loose teeth, deafness or loss of hearing. May have copious, clear urination or night urination or dribbling urination, incontinence, insufficient urine, oedema, runny stools, leukorrhea. The tongue will be swollen and pale with scallops on the sides and a moist, thin, white moss. The pulse will be frail and slow or minute and may be sinking in the Kidney position. The patient will show signs of general debilitation.

Deficiency of Yin of the Kidneys
The Kidney Water is exhausted with 'Empty Fire'.* The patient will look thin and shrivelled and will have a dry throat, hot palms and soles, red cheeks, afternoon fever or hot flushes, night sweats, reddish tongue with little moss. There may be ringing in the ears or loss of hearing with a weak sore back. A man may have little sperm and/or premature ejaculation. A woman may have a little vaginal secretion. The patient may suffer from forgetfulness, vertigo,

*Empty fire = 'Appearance of Heat where primary disorder is deficient water (Yin) = Fire Disorder of the Deficient Yang type.

sluggish thinking, dizziness, blurred vision, tinnitus, poor memory, hot, dark yellow urine, constipation, and possibly may have excessive sexual dreaming. The pulse will be thin and rapid.

Deficiency of Yin of the Kidneys can result from a long illness or from excessive sexual activity. In this condition, the Yin is not strong enough to warm the body, nor can it perform its function of separating clear from turbid fluids. Hence the symptoms of oliguria and other urinary problems. Excess body fluid retention will also result.

Deficiency of Kidney Qi
Sore and weak lumbar area and knee joints. Frequent urination, dribbling urine after urination, incontinence, nocturnal emission, infertility, shortness of breath, asthmatic breathing, thready pulse.

Deficiency of Kidney Jing
Yin and Yang are both deficient, so there will not be marked signs of heat or cold. Patient will show signs of premature ageing, with bad teeth, brittle bones, poor memory. In a younger person the signs would be slow physical or mental development. The effect of this condition on the patient's sexuality will differ according to the relative deficiency of Yin or Yang. If the Yang is more deficient than the Yin, there will be impotence and lack of sexual interest. If the Yin is more deficient than the Yang, there will be premature ejaculation or insufficient vaginal secretions.

What are the energetic functions of the Urinary Bladder?
Receives urine from the Kidney; temporarily stores the urine; excretes the urine from the body when a certain amount has accumulated.

Bladder Patterns

Normal Functions
The Bladder's function is aided by the Yang function of the Kidney.

It receives urine from the Kidney, temporarily stores urine and discharges urine from the body when a certain amount has accumulated.

Abnormal Function

Dysfunction of the bladder will manifest as problems of retention (inability to retain or inability to discharge) often associated with deficient or disturbed Kidney Yang.

Excess: Excess heat and dampness lead to 'Damp-Heat in the Bladder' with frequent and urgent, or scanty urination, dark urine, burning pain in the urethra, possible blood clots or stones, red tongue with yellow (possibly greasy) coating, fairly rapid, full pulse, possible fever, backache, dry mouth or thirst. This damp-heat may accumulate and crystallize, leading to 'sand' (stones) with sudden urinary obstruction, occasional violent stabbing pain in groin or back, blood in urine, normal tongue.

If turbid heat is obstructing the Bladder, there will be cloudy or murky substances in the urine.

Deficiency: Problems of Deficient Bladder Qi often accompany deficient Kidney Yang, as stated above, and can manifest as Cold disorder of the deficiency type, where Bladder and Kidney Yang functions are deficient. This can occur from excess sexual activity, overwork and stress, prolonged illness, or after surgery.

Symptoms include: incontinence (often after surgery), or frequent urination or enuresis; dribbling urination, weak stream or retention; weakness of the lumbar region and knee joints; aversion to cold; pallor; moist, white tongue coating; thready, deep (frail) pulse.

Common Disorders of Water

1. Vertigo (deficient Yin of Kidney with Rising Liver Fire).
2. Lumbago
   (a) Cold-Dampness in Bladder and Du Mo = back pain, heavy head, headache, tight cervical region, deep pulse, thin, white tongue coating.
   (b) Deficiency of Kidney = slow onset, dull pain or ache, prolonged weak feeling in kidney region (often patients respond to question 'Do you have pain in the kidney region?' by saying 'no', but palpation makes them recall this dull, weak or achy feeling; especially men over 30). This sort of ache gets worse

when tired, better with rest, worse after sex (subtle), weak knees and thighs. Back doesn't go out.

Deficient Kidney Yang will be accompanied by pain or ache spreading to pelvic region (nonspecific prostatitis, etc.) from G.V.4, empty, weak or deep, racing pulse, moist, white tongue coat.

Deficient Kidney Yin will be accompanied by dull achy lumbago, uneasiness (uncontrolled Yang of Liver and Heart), insomnia, dry mouth, red tongue, rapid pulse.

3. Urinary incontinence/retention (see Bladder Syndromes, above).
4. Tinnitus (deficient Kidney Yin with Rising Liver Fire).

Note
Deficient Yin of Kidneys = hyperactive adrenals, hyperthyroidism, hypertension, insomnia, heart palpitations, vision and ears disturbed. Deficient Yang of Kidneys = adrenal hypoactivity, hypothyroidism, palpitations with oedema, chronic enteritis, nephritis, asthma, emphysema, cardiac insufficiency.

Wood Patterns (Liver/Gall-Bladder)

Before reading the pages that follow, close the book and write down correspondences to answer question 1, then list normal functions for each Zang–Fu, with abnormal functions that would occur if the organ or bowel's normal functions break down. Then open the book and check your answers.

1. **What do you know about Wood? (What are its correspondences?)**

2. **What are the energetic functions of the Liver?**

Normal	*Abnormal*
1. Stores blood; regulates its volume.	1. Bleeding problems, anaemia, chronic hepatitis, deficient blood, menstrual irregularities, amenorrhoea, pale fingernails, weak spasms.

2. Maintains the patency of flow of Qi with smooth functioning of emotions, free flow of Qi through the other Zang–Fu bile secretion.

2. Constrained Liver Qi with purple tongue, wiry pulse, anger and depression, blocked throat, cystic or painful breasts, neck and groin. Lumps, dysmenorrhoea.

3. Controls the tendons. Yin of the Liver (Blood) nourishes the capacity of the tendons and muscles for movement.

3. Deficient Liver Yin = muscle spasms, dryness of the eyes or vision problems, wiry, nervous pulse, tension disorders, hypertension, menopausal emotional problems, etc.

4. The Liver opens to the eyes.

4. All hot, dry, blurry eye problems.

5. The Liver needs moisture from the Kidneys.

5. Liver Fire Blazing Upward (due to Constrained Liver Qi or dramatic emotional changes). Liver Fire Rising with insomnia, irritability, headaches, dizziness, red face and eyes, deafness or ringing in the ears.

Most common disorders of the Liver (As an exercise, write down what treatments you would use, and why, and check against the texts referred to in this volume.)

1. Nervous tension (Constrained Liver Qi);
2. Insomnia (Deficiency of Yin of the Kidneys and Liver leading to Rising Fire of the Liver);
3. Ulcerous Stomach with nausea, vomiting, belching, diarrhoea (Constrained Liver Qi attacking the Spleen);
4. Cystic breasts, dysmenorrhoea (Constrained Liver Qi);
5. Migraines (Excess Liver Yang);
6. Hypertension (Liver Fire Rising or Deficient Liver Yin);
7. Eye problems, including conjunctivitis and glaucoma (Deficient Liver Yin)
8. Ear problems such as tinnitis, labyrinthitis (Liver Fire Blazing Upward)

Gall-Bladder

What are its functions?

Normal	*Abnormal*
1. Stores and excretes bile. (Aids digestion)	1. Pain in sides, dark urine, nausea, vomiting, greasy tongue, heat signs, slippery pulse (Damp Heat of the GB) Also may include bitter taste and vomiting bitter fluids.
2. Very dependent on Liver, with which it is paired.	2. Same symptoms as Liver problems including GB symptoms mentioned above.
3. Rules decisions (Nei Jing)	3. Rash behaviour = excess Indecision = deficiency May include vertigo, timidity, unclear vision, wiry, thin pulse.

Five-Phase Energetics

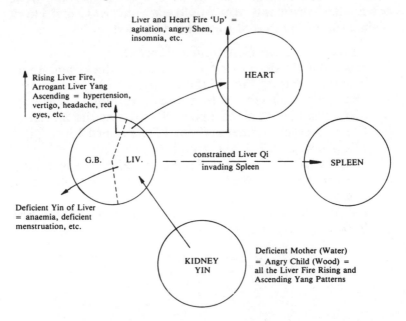

Liver and Heart Fire 'Up' = agitation, angry Shen, insomnia, etc.

Rising Liver Fire, Arrogant Liver Yang Ascending = hypertension, vertigo, headache, red eyes, etc.

HEART

G.B. / LIV.

constrained Liver Qi invading Spleen

SPLEEN

Deficient Yin of Liver = anaemia, deficient menstruation, etc.

KIDNEY YIN

Deficient Mother (Water) = Angry Child (Wood) = all the Liver Fire Rising and Ascending Yang Patterns

Common disorders of the Gall-Bladder: What treatments would you use and why?

1. Indigestion;
2. Headaches, especially on the sides of the head;
3. Sciatica, especially down the outside of the leg;
4. Flank pains.

Fire Patterns (Heart/Small Intestine; Pericardium/Triple Heater)

Reminder: Close your book and answer these questions. Then check against the book.

What do you know about Fire? (What are its correspondences?)

What does the Heart do?

Normal	Abnormal
1. Rules the Blood and Vessels.	1. Vessel and circulation problems.
2. Stores the Shen.	2. Disturbed Shen symptoms like insomnia, excess dreaming, forgetfulness, hysteria, irrationality, insanity, delirium.
3. Opens to the tongue.	3. Pale tongue = deficient blood; purple tongue = stagnant blood. Tongue inflammations and ulcer, talkativeness, slow speed, 'shaky' tongue.
4. Brilliance in the face.	4. Pale and lackluster complexion = deficient blood; red complexion = fire of the heart; purple complexion = stagnant heart blood.

What does the Pericardium do?

Normal	Abnormal
1. Protective shield of the heart. (The first line of defence against P.E. attacking the Heart.) Same as Heart.	1. Same as Heart. See above.

What does the Small Intestine do?

Normal	*Abnormal*
1. Separates pure from impure. Pure goes to the Spleen and impure to L.I.	1. Trouble with separation. Intestinal distress, malabsorption.

What does the Triple Heater do?

Normal	*Abnormal*
1. Controls the functional relationship between the organs that regulate water. (Lung, Spleen, Kidney)	1. Disturbed water and fluid metabolism (Oedema, etc.)
2. Upper Heater: Regulates breathing and circulation.	2. Respiratory distress and disorders of Heart and Lung associative pathways. Tight chest. Upper oedema.
3. Middle Heater: regulates digestion.	3. Digestive disturbances of the Liver effecting ST/Sp with swollen upper abdomen, middle oedema.
4. Lower Heater: regulates excretion.	4. Water in lower abdomen; excretory and urinary disorders, lower oedema.

Most common disorders: How would you treat them?

1. Deficient Heart Blood/Yin with heart palpitations, forgetfulness, insomnia, disturbed sleep, uneasiness. (The Blood/Yin cannot embrace Qi.) This may be associated with Deficient Spleen Qi (and Deficient Heart Blood) or Deficient Heart Yin and Deficient Kidney Yin, etc. (see chart).
2. Jueyin/Shaoyang (Wood–Fire) syndromes with all heart disorders and irregular beats, hypotension, hyperthyroid, sweating, migraines.
3. Taiyang/Shaoyin (Water–Fire) syndromes such as Hypertension, anaemia, hypothyroidism, constipation (Heart/S.I.), urinary retention.

Five-Phase Energetics (Fire)

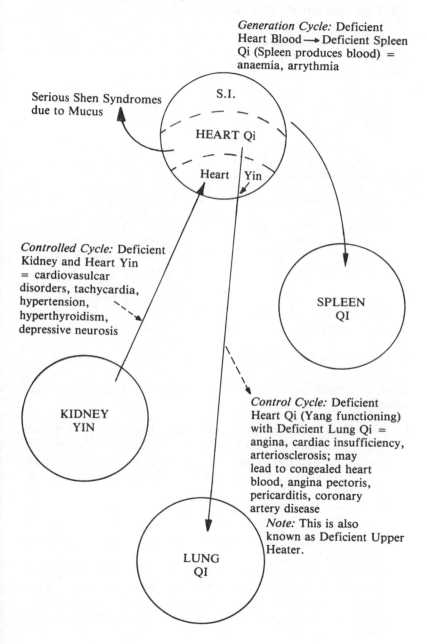

Generation Cycle: Deficient
Heart Blood → Deficient Spleen
Qi (Spleen produces blood) =
anaemia, arrythmia

Serious Shen Syndromes
due to Mucus

S.I.

HEART Qi

Heart Yin

Controlled Cycle: Deficient
Kidney and Heart Yin
= cardiovasulcar
disorders, tachycardia,
hypertension,
hyperthyroidism,
depressive neurosis

SPLEEN
QI

KIDNEY
YIN

Control Cycle: Deficient
Heart Qi (Yang functioning)
with Deficient Lung Qi =
angina, cardiac insufficiency,
arteriosclerosis; may
lead to congealed heart
blood, angina pectoris,
pericarditis, coronary
artery disease
    Note: This is also
known as Deficient Upper
Heater.

LUNG
QI

Earth Patterns (Stomach and Spleen)

What do you know about Earth?

What does the Spleen do?

Normal	*Abnormal*

1. Rules transportation and transformation. (Food is transformed to Qi, Blood, Ying and Wei.)
   (a) Sends Gu Qi (Grain Qi) up to Lungs (Taiyin) = synthesis of Qi and Blood.
   (b) Directs ascending movement.
   (c) Water movement and transformation.
	1. Deficient Qi and Blood Problems.
	
	   (a) Dropping organs (ptosis).
	   (b) & (c) Oedema, swollen abdomen.

2. Governs Blood (creates it and keeps it in the vessels).	2. Deficiency (anaemia), reckless blood (vomiting blood, blood in stools, bleeding under the skin, uterine bleeding).
3. Rules the flesh and muscles and extremities.	3. Atropy of the extremities, fleshiness obesity, sluggish limbs, fatigue.
4. Opens to the mouth and lips.	4. Loss of taste. Pale lips.

Most common disorders of the Spleen: What treatments would you use and why?

1. Deficient Spleen Qi with poor appetite, slight abdominal pain and distention relieved by pressure, pale tongue, scalloped tongue, empty pulse (Gastric and duodenal ulcers, dyspepsia of emotional origin, hepatitis, chronic dysentery, anaemia).
2. Deficient Spleen Yang. Like above but with more cold symptoms, cold limbs, watery stools with undigested food, oedema, difficulty urinating. (Ulcers, gastritis, dysentery).
3. Dampness of the Spleen which is like Deficient Yang with a soggy pulse, and thick greasy tongue moss and clogged head = nephritis (deficient Spleen and Kidney Yang).
4. Sinking Spleen Qi (ptosis) with haemorrhoids, prolapsed uterus, etc.

5. Spleen can't control the Blood with chronic bleeding (functional uterine bleeding), haemophilia, bleeding haemorrhoids.

What does the Stomach do?

Normal	*Abnormal*
1. 'Receives and ripens food and fluids'. Pure food goes to the Spleen (Biao–Li relationship) and impure goes to the S.I. (child–mother relationship).	1. Malabsorption.
2. Stomach rules 'descending'.	2. Nausea, vomiting, stomach ache, distention, belching, reflux oesophogitis.

Most common disorders of the Stomach: What treatments would you use and why?

1. Stomach Fire Rising with a rapid and full pulse.
2. Deficient Stomach Yin with a thin and rapid pulse.
3. Congealed Blood in the Stomach with possible ulcers, stabbing pain.

Five-Phase Energetics

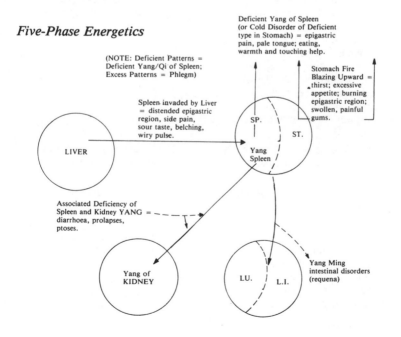

Deficient Yang of Spleen (or Cold Disorder of Deficient type in Stomach) = epigastric pain, pale tongue; eating, warmth and touching help.

(NOTE: Deficient Patterns = Deficient Yang/Qi of Spleen; Excess Patterns = Phlegm)

Stomach Fire Blazing Upward = thirst; excessive appetite; burning epigastric region; swollen, painful gums.

Spleen invaded by Liver = distended epigastric region, side pain, sour taste, belching, wiry pulse.

SP.

ST.

LIVER

Yang Spleen

Associated Deficiency of Spleen and Kidney YANG = diarrhoea, prolapses, ptoses.

Yang of KIDNEY

LU.

L.I.

Yang Ming intestinal disorders (requena)

Metal Patterns (Lung and Large Intestine)

What do you know about Metal? (What are its correspondences?)

What do the Lungs do?

Normal

1. The 'tender organ' (most easily effected by P.E.).

2. 'Rule Qi'. The 'foundation of Qi. Regulate the whole body Qi. Administer respiration.

3. Inhalation — take in air — descending function. Exhalation — expel impure air — disseminating function.

4. Closely related to 'Chest Qi' which moves the Qi and Blood in the body.

5. Move and adjust the Water channels. The upper origin of water: Descending — Lungs liquify water vapour and move it to Kidney/Bladder. Disseminating — circulates and scatters water vapour throughout the body, especially skin and pores (vapour form circulates or ascends).

6. Rule the exterior of the body — skin, body hair, sweat glands.

7. Wei Qi depends on the Lungs' disseminating function.

8. Open into the Nose, which is the 'thoroughfare for respiration'. Throat is the 'door of the Lungs', and the throat is the 'home of the vocal cords'.

Abnormal

1. Wind or wind/heat disorders with phlegm and mucus.

2. Weakness, tiredness.

3. Breathing problems with dyspnoea, asthma, irregular breathing, cough, chest distention.

4. Deficient Qi or Stagnant Qi anywhere.

5. Sweating problems, oedema of upper body, urinary problems.

6. Dry skin, excessive sweat, lowers resistance to P.E.

7. Getting sick easily with colds or whatever sickness is 'around'.

8. Nose and throat disorders; voice problems.

What do the Large Intestines do?

Normal	*Abnormal*
1. Move turbid parts of food and fluid down.	1, 2 Problems with defecating — & 3. diarrhoea or constipation (loose or dry stools, unformed stools, etc. Intestinal rumblings, abdominal pain.
2. Absorb water from waste material.	
3. Form and eliminate faeces.	

Most common disorders of Metal: What treatments would you use and why?

Lung
1. Coughing
   (a) Caused by P.E. with yellow tongue coat if heat, white, if cold.
   (b) Internal causes of coughing, including deficiency of Spleen (mother) due to dampness, phlegm (sticky cough) and Fire coming from the Liver (impinging back on metal) with bouts of coughing, red complexion, dry mouth. (In Western Medicine = Bronchitis, asthma, etc.)
2. Emphysema wherein the Kidney Yang is down and can't grasp the Qi.

Large Intestine
Constipation
1. Deficiency (emptiness) with sallow complexion, whitish nails, headaches and heart palpitations (rising energy) physical debility, white pale tongue coat.
2. Excess (fullness) moving the bowels only every 3–5 days, difficulty defecating, feeling hot, red complexion, thirst and other head symptoms.

Five-Phase Energetics

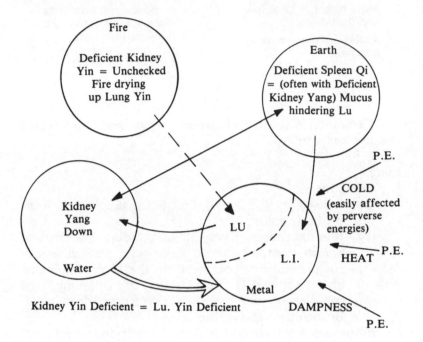

4.
AN EXAMPLE

Let us take a case and work through the energetic diagnosis, step by step according to the approach delineated above.

Case

A male patient 36 years old comes to you complaining of ringing in the ears, dizziness and a feeling of weakness.

Upon observation, the physician notes a red tongue with no coating and that the patient sits slumped at the waist. Listening uncovers mild productive coughing and a weak voice. Inquiry reveals a minor amount of hearing loss over the past six or seven years, a chronic tendency to fainting, a feeling of heat while sleeping and occasional night sweats for the past several years. Palpation indicates weakness in the area of the kidneys and evaluation of the pulses reveals a weak, thin, rapid pulse.

Steps

1. Differentiation of signs and symptoms

Feeling of weakness: weakness, deficiency.

Ringing in the ears: weakness, rising energy, possible Liver or Kidney sphere involvement.

Dizziness: energetic weakness or blood deficiency.

Red tongue: internal heat.

Slumped posture: weak lumbar region.

Productive cough: possible lung involvement (cold).

Weak voice: deficiency.

Hearing loss: deficiency, possible Kidney sphere involvement.

Slow development of present disharmony over at least seven years: chronic.

Night heat: deficiency of Yin.

Night sweats: deficiency.

Weakness in kidney region: possible Kidney sphere involvement.

Weak, thin, rapid pulse: deficiency with heat.

2. Presence of pernicious influences
No indication exists of the presence, in this disharmony, of exogenous factors, since the pulse is not floating and the history does not indicate this.

3. Is this a disorder of Zang-Fu or the meridians? Which ones?
This is clearly a Zang disturbance with possible involvement of the energetic spheres of the Kidneys, Liver and perhaps, Lungs, with Kidney imbalance predominating.

4. Evaluation according to the Eight Guiding Criteria
The disorder appears to be Internal, Deficient and Yin with a presence of Heat.

5. Working diagnosis
All data leads to a diagnosis of deficiency of Yin of the Kidneys with possible rising Liver Yang.

6. Treatment principle
Build Yin of the Kidneys and tend to the Rising Yang (branches).

7. Treatment strategy
Use local and distal points from the Kidney meridian; Use Mu and Shu points from the Liver and Kidney spheres; tonify the Yin of the Kidney and promote smooth functioning of the Liver sphere.

8. Selection of methods
Use acupuncture. Moxibustion is contraindicated in deficient Yin.

9. Selection of points

Kidney 7 and 10 to tonify the Yin of the Kidneys (Water and Tonification points) as the key distal points. Liver 3 may be chosen to promote smooth functioning of the Liver sphere if tonification of Kidney Yin is not sufficient.

Bladder 23 and G.B. 25 (Mu and Shu points of the Kidney sphere).

Conception Vessel 4 and 6: to build Kidney Qi in general.

Van Nghi suggests the addition of the Extra Point on the left side (3 Cun lateral to C.V. 4; the left side = Kidney Yin, the right side = Kidney Yang).

Next steps

If the above treatment helps with the low energy but is not sufficient to deal with the dizziness and tinnitus, one might suspect more important involvement of the Liver sphere, specifically deficient Yin of the Liver leading to Rising Yang symptoms. One could then add the Mu and Shu points of the Liver sphere (BL 18 and Liver 14), Liver 3, Gall-Bladder 20 from the Paired Fu sphere for dizziness, and Triple Heater local and distal points (T.H. 17, T.H. 5) for the tinnitus, through its association not only with the ear but with the Gall-Bladder Meridian (Shaoyang).

Comments

The above procedure guided us ever more clearly towards the affected organ energetic sphere. Let us now explain in more theoretical terms what the disorder is. In deficient Yin of the Kidneys, there will often be deficiency of Yin of the Liver (weak Mother unable to nourish the Child). Five-Phase rationale is built into this pattern. To pursue, if the Yin of the Liver sphere is deficient, it will not be sufficient to control the Yang (Gall-Bladder), giving rise to unchecked Wood Yang energy which invades the Liver channel. Yang energy tends to move upward, often as heat, whence the dizziness and tinnitus and red tongue, as well as the tendency to fainting.

It should be noted that deficiency of Yin of the Kidney can also lead to deficiency of all Yin, leading to uncontrolled Yang (Fire) of the Heart. The symptoms would include insomnia and uneasy feelings in the region of the heart. If this grows worse, the destruction cycle will be activated, and the

Fire will attack Metal, namely producing a deficiency of Lung Qi with dry cough, cold sweats and possible coughing up of blood.

5.
SELECTING TREATMENT STRATEGIES

Once a treatment principle has been selected according to the procedure outlined in Chapter 2, strategies must be selected appropriate to the treatment principle. The current texts on Traditional Chinese Medicine are very vague in this area, rarely doing more than providing a formula of points for a specific disorder or energetic imbalance. If one looks carefully, it becomes clearer that there are recurrent types of strategies chosen, and patterns of organizing a treatment plan. What follows is a summary of the most common treatment strategies and indications for their use in the treatment of internal energetic disturbances of the energetic orbs (Zang–Fu) of Chinese medicine. For a thorough discussion of energetic treatment of external disturbances of the tendino-muscular meridians and secondary vessels of acupuncture, the reader is referred to the excellent text by Royston Low, *Secondary Vessels of Acupunture*. In this text, Low provides a detailed discussion of the major work of Dr Nguyen Van Nghi on the treatment of the secondary vessels, along with a critical appraisal of these theories in the light of his own clinical experience.

Before enumerating common treatment strategies, it is important to keep in mind the overriding treatment principle of acupuncture, namely to treat the 'branches' (acute symptoms and conditions) in a sudden or acute condition, moving on to a treatment of the 'root' (energetic imbalance underlying the presenting complaint) when the acute symptoms have been pacified. In the case of a chronic disorder, treatment is generally directed at the root, with treatment of presenting symptoms and complaints occupying a secondary place in the treatment plan.

Another crucial point in sophisticated energetic treatment by acupuncture therapy involves the treatment by opposite polarities (Yin by Yang, Upper by Lower, Right by Left, etc.). In treating an energetic disturbance of the Liver orb, as an example, in addition to selecting local and distal points of the Liver meridian (Foot Jueyin) itself, one might select from the following:

1. the Liver orb's paired orb (internally/externally), namely the Gall-Bladder meridian (Foot Shaoyang);
2. the Great meridian at the opposite polarity, in this case, Hand Jueyin, namely the Pericardium meridian (known as treating Lower by Upper);
3. the orb in question's great meridian's paired great meridian, namely treating Shaoyang (Gall-Bladder and Triple Heater) for a disorder of Liver (which belongs to Jueyin, Liver and Pericardium, the pair to Shaoyang).

With these general principles in mind, let us look at some common treatment strategies.

A. Strategy of Local-Distal Points*

The major *local points* are points, in the area of dysfunction, that regulate function, namely the *Mu* and *Shu* points (alarm and associated effect points), points of the *three heaters* (upper heater = C.V. 17; middle heater = C.V. 11,12,13; lower heater = C.V. 3,4,6) and any other points in the affected zone that have a direct effect on corresponding functions (such as Kidney 27 for Kidney deficiency asthma, Bladder 31,32,33 for local pelvic complaints, etc.).

The major *distal points* are: the Five element points (command points); the Five Shu points (Jing-Well, Rong Spring, Shu-Stream, Jing-River, He-Sea); Source-Luo points; Xi (Cleft) points. These points and their usage constitute separate treatment strategies in and of themselves, and will be discussed in the following pages.

The method of using local-distal points is simple, and is outlined under the 'Excess' and 'Deficiency' headings below.

_____

*This strategy, as well as some of those to follow, are explained in somewhat different form in *Traite Didactique d'Acupuncture Traditionnelle*, by Andre Faubert, Guy Tredaniel Editors, Paris, 1977.

In excess conditions
Select more distal points, which are the main points to calm hyperactivity of an energetic orb. Use less local points, which are selected to direct the calming action of the distal points. Apply dispersing techniques to the distal points and neutral technique to the local points.

In deficiency conditions
Select more local points, which are the main points to tonify deficient energetic function. Apply tonification techniques to these points (warming techniques including moxibustion). Use less distal points and apply neutral techniques to these points, to harmonize the local tonifying action.

In my clinical experience over the past six years, this is by far the most common and overriding treatment strategy chosen for all disorders confronting an acupuncture therapist. All other treatment strategies are simply methods for selecting the most effective local or distal points for a given type of disorder and according to the therapist's orientation.

In brief, then, the choice of a local point orients the treatment strategy to the affected energetic functional sphere or zone (in internal energetic disturbances) while the distal points serve to determine the nature of the energetic manipulation (tonification, dispersal, warming, cooling, harmonizing, etc.). The combination of local and distal points forms a pattern of treatment that resembles the pattern of disharmony treated. In its most sophisticated application, a treatment pattern and its effects will confirm the diagnosis of the pattern of disharmony.

B.   Strategy of Mu–Shu Points

The Mu (Alarm) and Back Shu (Associated Effect) points are the most common local points utilized in the treatment of energetic disturbances of a functional orb. Generally speaking, the Mu points (Liver 13 for the Spleen, Conception 12 for the Stomach, etc.) are more specifically used for Yin disturbances of storing or depletion of energy reserves. The Back Shu points, on the other hand, are indicated in disturbances of Yang (function in general). In the case of a depletion of Yin in the Yin Zang, then, Liver 13 would be more specific than the Back Shu points for the Spleen, Liver and Kidney. Contrariwise, in a disturbance of Bladder function with dribbling urination, the Back Shu points of the Bladder and Kidney orbs are more appropriate than the Front Mu points. If one wishes to emphasize the treatment of the Yin or Yang aspect of an orb, this general principle is quite useful. However, in common clinical practice, this specificity is often avoided in favour of a more harmonizing strategy, namely that of utilizing both the Front Mu and Back Shu points together (either by applying the front or back points first, withdrawing them after a certain amount of time and then applying the points on the other body surface; or by treating back points for a period, alternated with front points).

One should note that in applying either the Mu or the Shu points, one can either tonify or disperse these points, depending on the condition (tonifying Liver 13 to increase Yin of the Spleen and Yin orbs in general; dispersing Conception Vessel 17 to disperse excess Yin/Fluids in the Lungs; tonifying Bladder 20 for deficiency of the Spleen orb's Yang function of transforming and transporting; dispersing Bl. 15 in a case of hyperactivity of the Heart orb or Heart Fire Blazing Upward, etc.).

C. Strategy of Source and Connecting (Luo) Points

In the case of internal/external disturbance within an element, one may select the source point of the Orb presenting the greatest difficulties, and the connecting (luo) point of the paired meridian. In the case of an internal/external imbalance in Metal, with constipation and asthma (Large Intestine and Lung) if one determines that the fundamental problem is a deficiency in the Lung Orb with a concommittant excess in the Large Intestine Orb, the treatment is as follows: select the source point of the Lung meridian and the connecting (luo) point of the paired, Large Intestine, meridian. This will serve to equalize the energy in the two paired Orbs.

Dr. Nguyen Van Nghi offers a clarification of the use of the source/luo points that has proven itself clinically in my own practice. Van Nghi states that in a deficiency, say of the Lung

Orb in this case, one must tonify the source point in order to draw the excess of energy from the Large Intestine to the Lung. In the case of an excess, one would disperse the source point, to allow for energy to move back to the relatively depleted Large Intestine Orb. Needling of the luo point in either case is generally neutral, but verging on dispersal, to 'disengage' the luo point and open it up.

Other authors and practitioners feel that it does not matter whether one chooses the source or the luo point of the most affected Orb, as the simple use of source and luo together is harmonizing. The clinician must determine in his own clinical experience which approach to this strategy works best for him.

D. Strategy of the Five Element and Five Shu Points

The Five Element (Wood, Fire, Earth, Metal and Water starting from the nail for Yin meridians; Metal, Water, Wood, Fire, Earth starting from the nail for Yang meridians) points are identical to the Five Shu points (Jing–Well, Rong–Spring, Shu–Stream, Jing–River, He–Sea). Hence the Jing–Well point of a Yin meridian is the Wood point. The Jing–Well point for a Yang meridian is the Metal point. Likewise, the He–Sea point of a Yin meridian is the Water point, and for a Yang meridian, the Earth point.

In utilizing these points, one must always be clear about which strategy one is adopting in selecting these points.

In using these points according to Five-Element theory, one may choose Water points to cool Fire, Fire points to disperse Water, etc. One may also use any of the many different strategies for manipulating energy along the generation and control cycles of the Five Phases. These different strategies all evolve out of the use of tonification and dispersal points and find their epitome in the different versions of the Four-Needle Technique.*

Tonification and dispersal points

To determine which is the *tonification point* for a meridian, one selects the Mother Element on the meridian in question.

*For a detailed discussion of these Five-Phase strategies, See Mary Austin, *Acupuncture Therapy*, and Kiko Matsumoto, *Five Elements, Ten Stems*, Redwing Books Boston, 1984.

In the case of the Lung meridian, for example, the Mother Element of the Lungs is Earth (Earth is the Mother of Metal). The tonification point of the Lung meridian would therefore be the Earth point on the Lung meridian, namely Lung 9. To determine the *dispersal point*, one selects the Child Element. In the case of the Lung meridian, the Child Element is Water (Water is the Child of Metal). The dispersal point of the Lung meridian would therefore be the Water point on the Lung meridian, namely Lung 5. The same principle holds true for all the other eleven regular meridians. Many people merely memorize these points, but it must be borne in mind that the use of tonification and dispersal points is a key Five-Element strategy, and that these points are best utilized in combination with other points according to Five-Element theory.

The Four-Needle technique
The Four-Needle technique makes use of tonification and dispersal points as well as points along the control cycle. There are many different versions of this technique, explored by Kiko Matsumoto in her fine work on the subject.* We will present the most common version utilized in the West.

In deficiences
Needle 1: Tonify the deficient meridian at its Mother (tonification) point. In the case of Lung deficiency, tonify the Earth point of the Lung, Lung 9.

Needle 2: Tonify the Master point on the Mother Element. In this case, the Mother of Metal is Earth, hence the Mother of Lung is Spleen. One tonifies the Master (Earth) point of the Spleen (Earth), namely Spleen 3.

Needle 3: Disperse the Controller Element on the affected meridian. In this case, the Controller of Metal is Fire, so one selects the Fire point on the affected meridian, the Lung, namely Lung 10.

Needle 4: Disperse the Master Point on the Controller Element. In this case, the Controller Element is Fire, hence the Controller of Lung is Heart. One disperses the Master (Fire) point on the Heart (Fire), namely Heart 8.

To summarize this principle for deficiency conditions:

*See previous footnote.

Tonify the first two needles:
1. Tonify the Mother element point on the affected meridian.
2. Tonify the Master point on the Mother Element itself.

Disperse the second two needles:
3. Disperse the Controller Element point on the affected meridian.
4. Disperse the Master point on the Controller Element.

In excesses

Needle 1: Disperse the Child Element point on the affected meridian. In the case of Spleen Excess, disperse the Metal (Child) point of the Spleen, namely the dispersal point Spleen 5.

Needle 2: Disperse the Master point on the Child meridian. In this case, the Child of Spleen is Lung. Disperse the Master (Metal) point of the Lung, Lung 8.

Needle 3: Tonify the Controller Element on the affected meridian. The Controller of Earth is Wood, so tonify the Wood point on the Spleen (Earth) meridian, namely Spleen 1.

Needle 4: Tonify the Master point on the Controller. The Controller in this case is Liver (Wood), so tonify the Master (Wood) point on the Liver, namely Liver 1.

To summarize this principle for excess conditions:

Disperse the first two needles:
1. Disperse the Child Element (Dispersal) point on the affected meridian.
2. Disperse the Master point on the Child meridian.

Tonify the second two needles:
3. Tonify the Controller Element on the affected meridian.
4. Tonify the Master point on the Controller meridian.

It should be noted that treatment by means of the Four-Needle technique is very powerful, and should only be initiated when a strong energetic manipulation is required, and only when one is certain of the primary element or Phase affected. The reasons for this should be obvious. The Four-Needle technique tonifies twice, then disperses twice, leading to a very concentrated tonifying or dispersing action on the affected element and meridian. If one is not certain of the primary element affected, it is far more judicious to use the more gentle tonification and dispersal points.

The Five Shu Points according to the seasons:
In question 74 of the *Nan–Ching* the following correspondence appears:

> In the Spring, needle the Jing–Well points.
> In the Summer, needle the Rong–Spring points.
> In the Late Summer, needle the Shu–Stream points.
> In the Fall, needle the Jing–River points.
> In the Winter, needle the He–Sea points.

While there are other interpretations of this use of the Five Shu points of command according to the seasons, this is a very common usage, and usually translates into a very common strategy: use Jing–Well points in acute situations (sudden, acute crises are like the Wind of Spring); use Jing–River points when the perverse energy has penetrated into the joints and become lodged there; use He–Sea points when a disorder has become internal and chronic, affecting the Sea of Energy, the 'Winter' of a disorder.

The Five Shu Points according to the level of attack:
In Chapter 6 of the *Ling Shu*, the following correspondence is given:

> In external disorders of Yang of Yang, use the Ahshi points.
> In external disorders of Yin of Yang, Use Jing–River points.
> In internal disorders of Yang of Yin, use He–Sea points.
> In internal disorders of Yin of Yin, use Rong–Spring and Shu–Stream points.

This passage is interpreted to mean:

External disorders
Yang of Yang = Skin, flesh, tendino-muscular meridians.
Yin of Yang = Muscles and bones.
Yang of Yin = Bowels (Fu, yang organs).
Yin of Yin = Organs (Zang, yin organs).
    This is a widely used strategy and a very good method for selecting strong distal points in a treatment plan.

Strategy E: Use of Xi-Cleft Points

This is a very common treatment strategy for selecting powerful distal points for acute disorders of a meridian and its Orb. One merely selects the Xi–Cleft point corresponding to the affected meridian/Orb. These points appear in all major textbooks of acupuncture and will not be repeated here.

Strategy F: Use of Common Points for Patterns of Qi, Xue (Blood), Jin Ye (Fluids)*

1. Energy Patterns

(a) *Qi Deficiency* (tonify Qi): Kid. 3, Bl. 23, G.V. 4, C.V. 4, Bl. 20 & 21, St. 36, Sp. 6, Liver 13, C.V. 17.

(b) *Fading Qi* (Qi Xian) (Build Qi and cause it to rise): C.V. 12, St. 25, G.V. 1, Bl. 35, C.V. 4 & 6.

(c) *Stagnant Qi* (circulate Qi): C.V. 12, C.V. 2, Sp. 6, St. 36, Liver 3, and painful points in stagnant zones.

2. Blood Patterns

(a) *Blood Deficiency* (fortify blood): Bl. 43, Bl. 20, Bl. 17, Sp. 10, St. 36

(b) *Congealed Blood* (fortify Qi to move the blood): Bl. 20 & 21, Sp. 6, St. 36, Liver 3, Sp. 1, Sp. 10, T.H. 3, St. 29.

(c) *Hot Blood* (Cool Down the Heat, Revive the Blood): Sp. 6 & 10, Liver 3, L.I. 4, Per. 6, Lung 9, Bl. 40(54)–Bleed.

3. Qi and Blood Patterns

(a) *Stagnant Qi with Congealed Blood* (Circulate Qi & Blood): G.V. 20, G.B. 20, G.B. 22, L.I. 4, Liver 3, Liver 13, Liver 14, T.H. 15, L.I. 13, St. 29.

(b) *Deficient Qi and Blood* (Strengthen Qi & Blood): G.V. 20, G.B. 20, Sp. 10, Bl. 43, L.I. 4, Sp. 6, St. 25.

(c) *Deficient Qi and Loss of Blood* (Strengthen Qi, Bring Blood Back into the Channels): Bl. 20 and 21, Sp. 6, St. 36, Sp. 10, Liver 3, C.V. 4 and 7.

4. Body Fluids (Jin Ye) Patterns

(a) *Deficiency of Body Fluids* (Increase fluids): Bl. 21, C.V. 12, Kid. 2 and 6, Sp. 6, Per. 8 (disperse).

(b) *Stagnant Body Fluids: Mucus* (Tan) *Stagnation:*
  (i) *Wind–Mucus* (chase wind, dissolve mucus): G.V. 26 and 22, S.I. 9, Liv. 14, G.B. 41, St. 40, Liver 3, G.B. 21, G.V. 11, G.V. 15.
  (ii) *Heat–Mucus* (disperse heat, dissolve mucus): L.I. 11, T.H. 5, Bl. 40 (54), Bl. 60, G.B. 34, G.V. 14, St. 40, G.V. 10, Kid. 8.
  (iii) *Cold–Mucus* (dissolve mucus through warming methods): C.V. 4 and 6 (moxa), G.V. 4 (moxa), Bl. 23, Kid. 3, C.V. 12.
  (iv) *Damp–Mucus* (Dry the Dampness, dissolve mucus): C.V. 9, Sp. 9, St. 40, Lu. 5, C.V. 4 and 12, Bl. 20 and 51, G.B. 28.
  (v) *Dry–Dampness* (moisten the dryness and dissolve the mucus): Bl. 13; C.V. 22, 17 and 14; S.I. 15; Lu. 1, 7 and 9; St. 15.
(c) *Yin (Phlegm) Patterns*
  Tan Yin in Stomach (warm the body and dissolve the Tan Yin): C.V. 12, Bl. 20 and 21, Sp. 17, Per. 6, St. 36, St. 40.
(d) *Oedema Patterns (Shui Qi or Shui Zhong)*
  (i) FULLNESS OEDEMA:
    – *External Pathogenic Wind* (Liberate Diffusing Function of the Lungs, Cause Water to Circulate): Bl. 13, Lu. 7, L.I. 4, G.V. 26.
    – *Water–Dampness* (Circulate Yang and Water): C.V. 9, C.V. 3 & 2, St. 28, Kid. 5, Kid. 7, Sp. 9.
    – *Damp–Heat Stagnation* (Cool the Heat and cause dampness and phlegm to circulate): C.V. 9, C.V. 6, Bl. 11 & 22, St. 36, Sp. 6, L.I. 4.
  (ii) DEFICIENCY OEDEMA
    – *Yang of the Spleen not Circulating* (Strengthen the Spleen's transformation and transportation functions, circulate water): Bl. 20, Liver 13, St. 36, Sp. 6, G.B. 41.
    – *Deficient Yang of the Kidney* (Warm Kidney Yang and Circulate Water): Bl. 20 & 23, C.V. 8, C.V. 4, St. 36 (moxa on all those preceding points), Sp. 6.

Note: In utilizing these general points for patterns of excess or deficiency of Qi, Blood or Fluids, it is essential to see these as adjunctive combinations only, to be added to local and distal points of the appropriate meridian or organ-energetic-system (Zang–Fu).

Summarized from Auteroche and Navail, *Le Diagnostic en Medecine Chinoise*, Maloine Publishers, Paris, 1983, pp.233–53).

Final Note on the Selection of Treatment Strategies

The Chinese texts do not explain how to use treatment strategies in any significant detail because points are often selected by their energetic action, which the Chinese practitioner will have memorized. I have found that the teaching and learning of acupuncture points by memorizing their individual function confuses students and leads to a very stereotyped kind of treatment that leaves no room for the personal development of the acupuncture therapist. It seems to me that a dedicated practitioner should work toward a level where he selects points and point combinations based on an almost intuitive sense that those particular points 'fit' the pattern of disharmony, 'confirm' the energetic diagnosis and are appropriate for the action selected by the acupuncture therapist. To develop a feeling for points and their usage, it is far wiser, I feel, to concentrate on the underlying strategies that determine what will be the effect of any particular group of points. In short, I feel that it is better for a therapist to select Lung 11 for swollen glands not because he memorized swollen glands as one indication for the point, but rather because he feels at home with the strategy of utilizing Jing–Well points in the Spring of a disorder, when symptoms flare up like a sudden gust of wind. Perhaps this is what Professor J. R. Worsley has in mind when he speaks of the role of 'intention' in selecting and manipulating acupuncture points. Rote-learning will never lead to a deep sense of intentionality in selecting appropriate treatments. An understanding of basic principles and strategies, and years of clinical experience, combined with a strong desire to learn to be at one with the person we treat, might at least point us in the right direction.
A good exercise to learn these strategies is to take the

disorders and treatments given in the back of the *Essentials of Chinese Acupuncture* and *Acupuncture: A Comprehensive Text*, and try to determine which strategies are being selected in the choice of points. The reader will be quite surprised to find that the strategies enumerated in the preceding pages are the most common strategies selected in these formula treatments. This will give one a different perspective on these treatment formulas. I believe that, just as the patterns of disharmony of the Zang–Fu, Qi, Blood and Fluids of Chinese medicine are not pure clinical realities, but rather pictures against which to measure the disturbances our clients present us with (as Kaptchuk clarifies in *The Web that has no Weaver*), so too the formulas given in texts such as those mentioned above are not recipes to be followed blindly, but 'images' of possible treatments to guide us in planning a treatment.

6.
EXERCISES TO LEARN THE APPROACH

In order to assess whether you have internalized this problem-solving process, try to use the nine-step procedure on the following three cases. Only when you are finished go to pages 226–31 of Kaptchuk's *The Web that has no Weaver* and see how well you did.

Case 1

The patient is a female graduate student with a lot of tension lately associated with studying for the past nine months for doctoral examinations. She complains of violent headaches, occasional dizziness, ringing in the ears and a dry mouth. Examination reveals a red face and red eyes. Upon questioning, she admits to frequent outbursts of anger and appears easily irritated. Recently she has been experiencing insomnia. She is a bit constipated and on palpation her pulse is rapid, full and wiry.

Case 2

A woman in her forties comes to you complaining of visual disturbances, especially very dry eyes and clouded vision. She has a slight tendency to hypertension and her physician has told her this is all 'just menopause'. He has prescribed Valium, which just makes her feel more agitated, especially before bed when it prevents her from falling asleep. Observation reveals reddish cheeks and nervousness. She states in the history that she sometimes gets dizzy and that she feels some internal heat in her palms and soles of the feet, and her pulse is wiry, rapid and thin.

Case 3

A man in his fifties comes to you with a diagnosis of hypertension. He periodically feels hot in his face and head, joking that perhaps he 'is going through the change of life'. He has frequent throbbing headaches, some pain in his eyes and they appear, on observation, to be a bit red. His history reveals some dizziness at times, and depression alternating with anger. Palpation reveals a wiry, rapid pulse.

Questions

Once you have worked through each of these three examples and feel satisfied with your assessments, and *before turning to Kaptchuk's book*, try to answer the following questions:

1. In case 1, how do you explain the insomnia, and the fact that the pulse is both rapid and wiry?
2. In case 2, how do you explain the three pulse qualities and the red cheeks?
3. In case 3, what are the throbbing headaches due to?

Now, turn to Kaptchuk's book and check your answers.

7.
WORKBOOK: CLINICAL CASES OF ZANG-FU PATHOLOGY

Introduction to Clinical Cases

In the cases that follow, you will note that a different number of steps from the nine-step problem-solving approach is requested every four to five cases, first requiring you to work through only step 1, then steps 1 and 2, and so forth, until you reach the second half of the cases, where you will be asked to work through all nine steps. This is in order to demonstrate the utility of a more detailed approach and also to reinforce and facilitate learning the nine steps one after the other.

Finally, the cases end with a 'self-check' referring you to page numbers in two key acupuncture texts. Be sure to check your responses, thereby reinforcing the learning experience.

It might be best for the reader to write down his responses to each part in the cases that follow on his own paper, then check responses against the pages in the 'self-check', finally writing the corrected responses in the book itself for future reference.

Case 1: Mary Jones

A child of 10 came in with her mother today complaining of itchy throat and cough with a watery nasal discharge. The child was slightly feverish with chills. She had spent the weekend playing out in the snow and today, being Monday, had woken up too sick to go to school. Her mother says, 'Whenever she has a test in arithmetic she gets sick, I just don't know what to do with her. Perhaps its psychological, doctor, what do you think? Her therapist says that she is insecure.'

1. Differentiation of signs and symptoms:

Note: To do a self-check, see *Essentials*, pp. 70–1, *The Web*, pp. 206, 217–20.

Case 2: Joseph Rollo

A 63-year-old man comes into the clinic. He complains of pains in his upper abdomen, especially on the sides. He says that he is used to 'enjoying an excellent digestion' and in fact, rich foods and wine are some of his favourite things. The practitioner notices that his facial colour and sclera both have a bright yellow cast; his tongue has a sticky yellow coating. The patient says that occasionally when he is feeling especially poorly, he vomits a sour, greenish fluid.

1. Differentiation of signs and symptoms:

Note: To self-check, see *Essentials*, pp. 73, *The Web*, pp. 278.

INNER TRADITIONS

BEAR & CO.

HEALING ARTS PRESS

DESTINY BOOKS

Park Street Press

BINDU BOOKS

BEAR CUB BOOKS

Please send us this card to receive our latest catalog.

☐ Check here if you would like to receive our catalog via e-mail.

E-mail address _____

Name _____ Company _____

Address _____

City _____ State _____ Zip _____ Country _____

Phone _____

Order at 1-800-246-8648 • Fax (802) 767-3726

E-mail: orders@InnerTraditions.com • Web site: www.InnerTraditions.com

Inner Traditions • Bear & Company
P.O. Box 388
Rochester, VT 05767-0388
U.S.A.

Case 3: Jim Sanchez

The patient has rumbling in the intestines with a painful abdomen, and some diarrhoea. Upon questioning the patient says that his urine is clear in colour. The tongue is moist with a greasy white coating. The pulse is deep and slippery.

1. Differentiation of signs and symptoms:

Note: To self-check, see *Essentials* pp. 74–5, *The Web*, pp. 223, 277–8.

Case 4: Susan Cohen

The patient complains of a 'bunch of problems'. She has a sore throat and also has a sore in her mouth. Her urination is frequent and slightly painful. The urine is dark. Her abdomen is slightly bloated. As she speaks the practitioner notes a pervading irritability in her manner. Her tongue is red with yellow coating; her pulse is rapid and slippery.

1. Differentiation of signs and symptoms:

Note: To self-check, see *Essentials*, p. 73, *The Web*, p. 212–13.

Case 5: Adrienne Jones

Today, the mother of the 10-year-old girl we saw last week came in without her daughter. The daughter, apparently is fine, but the mother now feels a cough with shortness of breath and she is bringing up a great deal of white frothy sputum. Her tongue coating is white and slightly sticky. She is a smoker and likes sweets as well.

1. Differentiation of signs and symptoms:

2. Determination of the presence or absence of exogenous pathogenic factors:

Note: To self-check see *Essentials,* p. 70, *The Web,* p. 218.

Case 6: Sam Chong

A 32-year-old man comes to the clinic complaining of violent pain in his abdomen. He says he is constipated and although he feels the urge, he cannot pass gas either. He says that he has vomited up some faecal matter. His tongue is greasy with a yellow coating; his pulse is wiry and full.

1. Differentiation of signs and symptoms:

2. Determination of the presence or absence of exogenous pathogenic factors:

Note: To self-check, see *Essentials*, p. 73, *The Web*, p. 277.

Case 7: Karen Reinhardt

A 25-year-old woman comes into the clinic complaining of pain on urination. She says that she has been feeling an urgent need to urinate, every couple of hours. When she urinates she has a burning pain and the urine does not come out smoothly. Upon questioning, she says that the urine is reddish in colour and that there is only a little, each time she goes. The practitioner notes that her tongue is reddish in colour with a yellow coating. Her pulse is slightly rapid.

1. Differentiation of signs and symptoms:

2. Determination of the presence or absence of exogenous pathogenic factors:

Note: To self-check see *Essentials*, p. 75, *The Web*, p. 279.

Case 8: Susan Allman

A 34-year-old woman comes into the clinic. She says that she suffers from a slight, persistent pain in her stomach. She says that when she uses a hot water bottle, it helps make the pain go away. When asked about her eating habits she says that she usually eats a lot of salad, but that lately she has been eating mostly soup which seems to help to make her feel better. Upon examination the practitioner finds she has a pale tongue with moist white coating. The pulse is deep and without strength.

1. Differentiation of signs and symptoms:

2. Determination of the presence or absence of exogenous pathogenic factors:

Note: To self-check see *Essentials*, p. 73, *The Web*, pp. 221–2.

Case 9: Thomas Callahan

A 50-year-old man comes into the clinic complaining of pain in his testicles. He says that he also feels some discomfort in the lower abdomen. Upon examination it is found that he has a pale tongue with white coating and a deep, slow pulse. During the history-taking he mentions that he is a member of the Polar Bear Club and also that he and his wife are separated.

1. Differentiation of signs and symptoms:

2. Determination of the presence or absence of exogenous pathogenic factors:

3. Determination of whether the disturbance is of the Zang–Fu or the meridians:

Note: To self-check see *Essentials*, p. 67–8, *The Web*, pp. 232–4.

Case 10: Jimmy Nakasawa

A 25-year-old man comes into the clinic complaining that he feels cold all the time and he has a constant achiness in his lower back. Upon further questioning, it is found that he suffers from dribbling urination and that he finds himself urinating more frequently than usual. His pulse is slightly slow, and his tongue has a thin white coating.

1. Differentiation of signs and symptoms:

2. Determination of the presence or absence of exogenous pathogenic factors:

3. Determination of whether the disturbance is of the Zang–Fu or the meridians:

Note: To self-check see *Essentials*, p. 75–6, *The Web*, p. 279.

Case 11: Richard Spatz

A patient complains of slight but persistent pain in the lower abdomen. His stools are watery and his abdomen is always gurgling. His tongue is pale with a thin white moss. The pulse is empty.

1. Differentiation of signs and symptoms:

2. Determination of the presence or absence of exogenous pathogenic factors:

3. Determination of whether the disturbance is of the Zang-Fu or the meridians:

Note: To self-check see *Essentials*, p. 73, *The Web*, pp. 221–2, 277.

Case 12: Adrienne Jones

It has been a month now since Mrs X, mother of the 10-year-old girl, first came to the clinic to be treated for her cough, etc. Although she feels better after treatment the cough and shortness of breath keep coming back and her sputum, although smaller in quantity, is now yellowish-green. She says that she is trying to stop smoking, but 'it's very difficult', and she is trying to cut down on eating so much sugar because she knows it isn't good for her. Still, she says, it's hard to discipline herself, especially since 'things' have been so problematic lately. Upon questioning, Mrs X mentions that although it is already the beginning of December, the landlord has not yet fixed the boiler and they have no heat in their home.

1. Differentiation of signs and symptoms:

2. Determination of the presence or absence of exogenous pathogenic factors:

3. Determination of whether the disturbance is of the Zang–Fu or the meridians:

Note: To self-check see *Essentials*, p. 70–1, *The Web*, pp. 206, 217–18.

Case 13: Ruth Feinberg

This is a 35-year-old woman who comes to the clinic because she is suffering from insomnia. A friend told her to try acupuncture. She is in the midst of finishing up a doctoral dissertation and has a lot of work she has to get done in the next two weeks. She is worried that loss of sleep is making it difficult for her to concentrate. She has tried sleeping pills but they don't really help and just make her feel drowsy and unable to concentrate all the more. She says, 'If acupuncture is going to make me feel that way, I don't want it.' She has some sores in her mouth 'from drinking too much coffee'. She looks flushed, almost feverish and upon questioning it is found that her urine is slightly darker than normal and that she has a bitter taste in her mouth sometimes. The practitioner finds her tongue is red; her pulse, rapid.

1. Differentiation of signs and symptoms:

2. Determination of the presence or absence of exogenous pathogenic factors:

3. Determination of whether the disturbance is of the Zang–Fu or the meridians:

4. Eight Guiding Criteria evaluation of the clinical data:

Note: To self-check see *Essentials*, p. 67, *The Web*, pp. 212, 213.

Case 14: Regina Lim

A 31-year-old woman comes to the clinic. She has constipation with dry stool. From the history, the practitioner finds out that she has recently given birth to a child. Her tongue is red and dry. The pulse is thin.

1. Differentiation of signs and symptoms:

2. Determination of the presence or absence of exogenous pathogenic factors:

3. Determination of whether the disturbance is of the Zang–Fu or the meridians:

4. Eight Guiding Criteria evaluation of the clinical data:

Note: To self-check see *Essentials*, pp. 74–5, *The Web*, pp. 277–8.

Case 15: Rita Haaz

A 30-year-old woman comes into the clinic complaining of feeling bloated in her abdomen and breasts. Her history shows that she works in a big department store and that store is in the midst of stocking up for the Christmas rush. She is busy. She says that occasionally she also feels 'as though something were stuck in her throat'. Upon questioning, it is noted that her periods have been somewhat irregular for the last few months as well. As she speaks, the practitioner also notices that she tends to sigh quite frequently.

1. Differentiation of signs and symptoms:

2. Determination of the presence or absence of exogenous pathogenic factors:

3. Determination of whether the disturbance is of the Zang–Fu or the meridians:

4. Eight Guiding Criteria evaluation of the clinical data:

Note: To self-check see *Essentials*, p. 67–8, *The Web*, pp. 226–7.

Case 16: Stuart Richardson

A 50-year-old man comes into the clinic. He has just recovered from a long illness and is on his feet again. However, he finds that, although the symptoms of his previous illness have cleared up, he still does not feel 'quite right'. He says that he always feels chilled and no matter what he wears, his hands and feet are always cold. His friends tell him he looks pale and he notices that when he climbs the stairs to his apartment he gets very short of breath and his heart 'flutters'.

Upon examination he is found to have a pale tongue and a thready pulse. His lips have a slightly purplish tinge and his face has an unhealthy pallor.

1. Differentiation of signs and symptoms:

2. Determination of the presence or absence of exogenous pathogenic factors:

3. Determination of whether the disturbance is of the Zan–Fu or the meridians:

4. Eight Guiding Criteria evaluation of the clinical data:

Note: To self-check see *Essentials*, pp. 65–6, *The Web*, pp. 213–14.

Case 17: Rick Lyman

This clinic is located in Phoenix, Arizona. It is July. A young man is brought into the clinic by his friends. They had been hiking in the dessert for the last few days when their friend developed a high fever and went into convulsions. His neck was rigid and his eyes bulging out. They would have taken him to the hospital, but the clinic was closer. Upon examination it is found that the young man has a deep-red tongue, a rapid and wiry pulse. His friends tell the practitioner that he has recently had a lot of problems at home since his father had to be hospitalized for a peptic ulcer and his mother was very worried.

1. Differentiation of signs and symptoms:

2. Determination of the presence or absence of exogenous pathogenic factors:

3. Determination of whether the disturbance is of the Zang–Fu or the meridians:

4. Eight Guiding Criteria evaluation of the clinical data:

5. Establishment of a working diagnosis:

Note: To self-check see *Essentials*, p. 67, *The Web*, p. 231.

Case 18: Sally Wright

A young woman comes into the clinic complaining of pain in her upper abdomen. She says that she is 'hungry and thirsty all the time'. When asked if she has any other medical problems, she says that she is going to the dentist tomorrow because her gums are swollen and sore. Upon examination she is found to have a reddish-coloured tongue with thick yellow coating. Her pulse is rapid and full.

1. Differentiation of signs and symptoms:

2. Determination of the presence or absence of exogenous pathogenic factors:

3. Determination of whether the disturbance is of the Zang–Fu or the meridians:

4. Eight Guiding Criteria Evaluation of the Clinical Data:

5. Establishment of a working diagnosis:

Note: To self-check see *Essentials*, pp. 73–4, *The Web*, p. 276.

Case 19: Tony Sims

A 40-year-old man comes into the clinic complaining that he is always cold and tired and wants acupuncture because his friend told him that it would 'give him more energy'. He insists that he feels fine except for this. Upon examination he is found to have a pale complexion, pale tongue and a deep and thready pulse. His legs get achy sometimes, he says, but that is because he works out several times a week on machines. He has no emotional problems to speak of, except, 'too many women and they all want to see me at the same time'.

1. Differentiation of signs and symptoms:

2. Determination of the presence or absence of exogenous pathogenic factors:

3. Determination of whether the disturbance is of the Zang–Fu or the meridians:

4. Eight Guiding Criteria evaluation of the clinical data:

5. Establishment of a working diagnosis:

6. Determination of the treatment principle:

7. Determination of the treatment strategy:

8. Selection of methods:

9. Selection of points: (Resource: to self-check, see *Essentials* pp. 71–2, *The Web* pp. 234–5.)

* Next steps:

Case 20: Nigel Thomas

A 45-year-old male patient comes into the clinic. He says that he has noticed pus in his stools. He says that when he has to defecate he feels a very urgent, sudden feeling to do so and that he also often feels a burning feeling in his anus. He thinks he may have a fever as well. The practitioner examines him and finds that his tongue is red with a greasy yellow coating. His pulse is slippery and rapid.

1. Differentiation of signs and symptoms:

2. Determination of the presence or absence of exogenous pathogenic factors:

3. Determination of whether the disturbance is of the Zang–Fu or the meridians:

4. Eight Guiding Criteria evaluation of the clinical data:

5. Establishment of a working diagnosis:

6. Determination of the treatment principle:

7. Determination of the treatment strategy:

8. Selection of methods:

9. Selection of points: (Resource: to self-check, see *Essentials* pp. 74–5, *The Web* pp. 277–8.)

* Next steps:

Case 21: Peter Carmichael

Today a vegan came into the clinic with 'stomach trouble'. He says he feels tired and heavy, especially his head and has no appetite. His health diet of raw vegetables and fruits does not interest him the way it usually does. He says that his chest and abdomen feel 'swollen' and there is a lot of noise coming from his abdomen. This young man cannot understand what the problem could be but he knows that it cannot be his diet because he is very careful to eat only the right foods. He says that he occasionally used to have stomach aches when he 'ate anything', but since he has converted to this diet (recommended by his guru) everything about his life and health have been perfect.

1. Differentiation of signs and symptoms:

2. Determination of the presence or absence of exogenous pathogenic factors:

3. Determination of whether the disturbance is of the Zang–Fu or the meridians:

4. Eight Guiding Criteria evaluation of the clinical data:

5. Establishment of a working diagnosis:

6. Determination of the treatment principle:

7. Determination of the treatment strategy:

8. Selection of methods:

9. Selection of points: (Resource: to self-check, see *Essentials* pp. 69–70, *The Web* pp. 223.)

* Next steps:

Case 22: Stuart Richardson (see also, case 16)

The 50-year-old male mentioned above decides that he really doesn't need treatment. He goes back to his high-powered executive job and resumes a ten-hour-day stressful schedule. Three months later he returns to the clinic complaining that he can't concentrate on his work anymore, he keeps forgetting his appointment schedule and he finds that he often breaks into a sweat for no reason at all. He is quite distressed. The practitioner finds that his pulse has become faded and thready.

1. Differentiation of signs and symptoms:

2. Determination of the presence or absence of exogenous pathogenic factors:

3. Determination of whether the disturbance is of the Zang–Fu or the meridians:

4. Eight Guiding Criteria evaluation of the clinical data:

5. Establishment of a working diagnosis:

6. Determination of the treatment principle:

7.   Determination of the treatment strategy:

8.   Selection of methods:

9.   Selection of points: (Resource: to self-check, see *Essentials* pp. 65–6, *The Web* pp. 213–14.)

* Next steps:

Case 23: Roslyn O'Reilly

A 28-year-old cocktail waitress comes into the clinic complaining of dizziness and feeling 'kind of out of it'. She says that she occasionally feels a hot sensation in her face and in her feet when she is working, and also, although she has been the top waitress at her place of employment for almost a year, lately she keeps forgetting which customers ordered what. She is quite concerned about all of this. Upon examination it is found that her tongue is red, her pulse thready and slightly rapid. Her urine is slightly darker red than usual. Her history reveals that she had been in bed for several months with hepatitis and has just gone back to work in the last two weeks.

1. Differentiation of signs and symptoms:

2. Determination of the presence or absence of exogenous pathogenic factors:

3. Determination of whether the disturbance is of the Zang–Fu or the meridians:

4. Eight Guiding Criteria evaluation of the clinical data:

5. Establishment of a working diagnosis:

6. Determination of the treatment principle:

7. Determination of the treatment strategy:

8. Selection of methods:

9. Selection of points (Resource: to self-check, see *Essentials* pp. 71–2, *The Web* pp. 235–6.)

* Next steps:

Case 24: Lionel Harvey

A 30-year-old graduate student comes to the clinic complaining of a 'stabbing' sensation in the 'stomach'. He says that pressure worsens the pain. His stools are very dark-coloured. The practitioner notices that his complexion is quite dark. His tongue is a dark red with red dots and a thin yellow coating. The pulse is wiry and choppy. He days that he does not, as a rule have stomach trouble, but that all this started just recently after he took a punch during karate class. 'Ever since then,' he says, 'I haven't felt quite right.'

1. Differentiation of signs and symptoms:

2. Determination of the presence or absence of exogenous pathogenic factors:

3. Determination of whether the disturbance is of the
    Zang–Fu or the meridians:

4. Eight Guiding Criteria evaluation of the clinical data:

5. Establishment of a working diagnosis:

6. Determination of the treatment principle:

7. Determination of the treatment strategy:

8. Selection of methods:

9. Selection of points (Resource: to self-check, see *Essentials* pp. 73–4, *The Web* pp. 276.)

* Next steps:

Case 25: Ralph Costello

A 60-year-old man comes to the clinic to 'quit smoking'. His grandson told him that acupuncture could really help him. He's tried to quit many times but 'old habits die hard' he says. 'How old a habit might that be, sir?' the practitioner asks him. 'Oh, about forty-five years, I guess.' The man has a dry cough which occasionally brings up thick mucus with specks of blood in it. His face is red and his mouth dry. Upon examination it is found that his tongue is red and his pulse thready and rapid. He says that occasionally he even wakes up in the middle of the night to have a cigarette. 'Sometimes it'll be 3 or 4 in the morning and I wake up drenched in sweat. Then I just have to have a cigarette to go back to sleep.'

1. Differentiation of signs and symptoms:

2. Determination of the presence or absence of exogenous pathogenic factors:

3. Determination of whether the disturbance is of the Zang–Fu or the meridians:

4. Eight Guiding Criteria evaluation of the clinical data:

5. Establishment of a working diagnosis:

6. Determination of the treatment principle:

7. Determination of the treatment strategy:

8. Selection of methods:

9. Selection of points (Resource: to self-check, see *Essentials* pp. 70–1, *The Web* pp. 218–19.)

* Next steps:

Case 26: Sam Jarvis

The patient feels an urgent pain in the right lower area of the abdomen and resists vehemently when the practitioner wants to press in the painful area. The tongue is red with yellow moss. The pulse is rapid.

1. Differentiation of signs and symptoms:

2. Determination of the presence or absence of exogenous pathogenic factors:

3. Determination of whether the disturbance is of the Zang–Fu or the meridians:

4. Eight Guiding Criteria evaluation of the clinical data:

5. Establishment of a working diagnosis:

6. Determination of the treatment principle:

7. Determination of the treatment strategy:

8. Selection of methods:

9. Selection of points (Resource: to self-check, see
    Essentials pp.74–5, *The Web* pp. 277–8.)

* Next steps:

Case 27: Nancy Sung

The patient comes to the clinic in very low spirits. She has chronic diarrhoea with a slight, but persistent lower abdominal discomfort. She says that her hands and feet are always cold. Her tongue is pale with a white moss. The pulse is frail.

1. Differentiation of signs and symptoms:

2. Determination of the presence or absence of exogenous pathogenic factors:

3. Determination of whether the disturbance is of the
    Zang–Fu or the meridians:

4. Eight Guiding Criteria evaluation of the clinical data:

5. Establishment of a working diagnosis:

6. Determination of the treatment principle:

7. Determination of the treatment strategy:

8. Selection of methods:

9. Selection of points (Resource: to self-check, see *Essentials* pp. 65-6, *The Web* pp. 277-8.)

* Next steps:

Case 28: Samuel Goldberg

A 42-year-old man comes into the clinic complaining of dizziness and headaches. He has a history of overindulgence in alcohol and smoking. His eyes and face are red. The practitioner finds his tongue is reddish with a yellow coating; his pulse rapid and wiry. The patient also complains 'I always have a bitter taste in my mouth, no matter what I eat.'

1. Differentiation of signs and symptoms:

2. Determination of the presence or absence of exogenous pathogenic factors:

3. Determination of whether the disturbance is of the Zang-Fu or the meridians:

4. Eight Guiding Criteria evaluation of the clinical data:

5. Establishment of a working diagnosis:

6. Determination of the treatment principle:

7. Determination of the treatment strategy:

8. Selection of methods:

9. Selection of points (Resource: to self-check, see *Essentials* pp. 67–8, *The Web* pp. 227–9.)

* Next steps:

Case 29: Jose Yamamoto

A man comes into the clinic complaining of an 'urgent pain' in the hypogastric area and the groin. He says that he has noticed that one of his testicles hangs lower than the other. The pain sometimes extends all the way to his lower back. His tongue has a white coating. His pulse is deep and wiry.

1. Differentiation of signs and symptoms:

2. Determination of the presence or absence of exogenous pathogenic factors:

3. Determination of whether the disturbance is of the Zang–Fu or the meridians:

4. Eight Guiding Criteria evaluation of the clinical data:

5. Establishment of a working diagnosis:

6. Determination of the treatment principle:

7. Determination of the treatment strategy:

8. Selection of methods:

9. Selection of points, (Resource: to self-check, see *Essentials* pp. 67–8, 73, *The Web* pp. 227, 232.)

* Next steps:

Case 30: Siva Saraswati

A mother brings in her 11-year-old daughter, complaining 'She eats like a bird,' and what she does eat, she doesn't keep down. The girl has a dry mouth and lips, with a peeled reddish tongue and a thin and rapid pulse. She says she doesn't eat because she isn't hungry.

1. Differentiation of signs and symptoms:

2. Determination of the presence or absence of exogenous pathogenic factors:

3. Determination of whether the disturbance is of the Zang–Fu or the meridians:

4. Eight Guiding Criteria evaluation of the clinical data:

5. Establishment of a working diagnosis:

6. Determination of the treatment principle:

7. Determination of the treatment strategy:

8. Selection of methods:

9. Selection of points (Resource: to self-check, see *Essentials* pp. 73–4, *The Web* pp. 276.)

* Next steps:

Case 31: Samson White

A 55-year-old man comes into the clinic, complaining of chest pain. He says that he had a heart attack five years ago. His doctor advised him to stop working so hard. Upon questioning the patient it is found that he has a high-pressure job in a big company. He also complains of pains in his upper back and shoulder which he says may be from sitting at a desk and talking on the telephone all day.

The practitioner examines him and finds his tongue is dark red — almost purple, as are his lips. The colour under his fingernails is dark. His pulse is thready, with occasional missed beats.

1. Differentiation of signs and symptoms:

2. Determination of the presence or absence of exogenous pathogenic factors:

3. Determination of whether the disturbance is of the Zang–Fu or the meridians:

4. Eight Guiding Criteria evaluation of the clinical data:

5. Establishment of a working diagnosis:

6. Determination of the treatment principle:

7. Determination of the treatment strategy:

8. Selection of methods:

9. Selection of points (Resource: to self-check, see *Essentials* pp. 65–6, *The Web* pp. 277–8.)

* Next steps:

Case 32: Maria MacDonald

A 16-year-old girl comes to the clinic complaining of loss of appetite and general tiredness. Her complexion is somewhat sallow and upon questioning, it is found that lately her stools are slightly loose. Her history includes a somewhat early onset of menstruation at age 10 and a broken leg at age 12. She is presently applying for college and hopes to qualify as one in 1,000 students competing for a scholarship.

1. Differentiation of signs and symptoms:

2. Determination of the presence or absence of exogenous pathogenic factors:

3. Determination of whether the disturbance is of the Zang–Fu or the meridians:

4. Eight Guiding Criteria evaluation of the clinical data:

5. Establishment of a working diagnosis:

6. Determination of the treatment principle:

7. Determination of the treatment strategy:

8. Selection of methods:

9. Selection of points (Resource: to self-check, see *Essentials* pp. 69–70, *The Web* pp. 221–2.)

* Next steps:

Case 33: Tomoko Kanai

A 17-year-old girl comes into the clinic complaining of feeling very weak and dizzy. She says that she suffers from a lot of pain in her arms and legs and that sometimes they even feel slightly numb. During the history-taking she tells the practitioner that she was recently in a serious car accident and was in the hospital for several weeks. She had a broken leg. She lost a great deal of blood and had to be given transfusions. Upon questioning she tells the practitioner that her menstrual flow is abnormally light-coloured and her cycle has increased from 30 to 40 days.

1. Differentiation of signs and symptoms:

2. Determination of the presence or absence of exogenous pathogenic factors:

3. Determination of whether the disturbance is of the Zang–Fu or the meridians:

4. Eight Guiding Criteria evaluation of the clinical data:

5. Establishment of a working diagnosis:

6. Determination of the treatment principle:

7. Determination of the treatment strategy:

8. Selection of methods:

9. Selection of points (Resource: to self-check, see *Essentials* pp. 67–8, *The Web* pp. 231–2.)

* Next steps:

Case 34: Ramona Santamaria

A 40-year-old woman comes into the clinic complaining of general restlessness and insomnia. Upon questioning her further it is found that she has recently recovered from a bad bout of influenza during which she had a high fever for about a week. She looks flushed and seems agitated. She says her heart feels funny sometimes and she also finds herself forgetting very simple things. She is quite worried and upset. She has been back at work for several weeks already and is finding that she can't keep up with her work like she used to because she feels so 'unsettled'.

Upon examination she is found to have a red tongue, and a thready and rapid pulse.

1. Differentiation of signs and symptoms:

2. Determination of the presence or absence of exogenous pathogenic factors:

3. Determination of whether the disturbance is of the Zang–Fu or the meridians:

4. Eight Guiding Criteria evaluation of the clinical data:

5. Establishment of a working diagnosis:

6. Determination of the treatment principle:

7. Determination of the treatment strategy:

8. Selection of methods:

9. Selection of points (Resource: to self-check, see
    Essentials pp.65–6, *The Web* pp. 212–13.)

* Next steps:

Case 35: Calhoun Alexander

A 55-year-old man comes into the clinic complaining of dribbling urination. He says that he has recently recovered from pneumonia and his doctor tells him that, although he should take it easy, he can begin to resume his regular activities. Concerning the problem of dribbling urination, the doctor said, 'Oh, don't worry about it.' Upon discussing his problems in more detail, it is found that he also suffers from occasional soreness in the lower back and shortness of breath which he attributes to his recent illness and having had to lie in bed for so long. His pulse is slightly thready.

1. Differentiation of signs and symptoms:

2. Determination of the presence or absence of exogenous pathogenic factors:

3. Determination of whether the disturbance is of the Zang–Fu or the meridians:

4. Eight Guiding Criteria evaluation of the clinical data:

5. Establishment of a working diagnosis:

6. Determination of the treatment principle:

7. Determination of the treatment strategy:

8. Selection of methods:

9. Selection of points (Resource: to self-check, see *Essentials* pp.71–2, *The Web* pp. 234–5.)

Case 36: Rose Smith

This patient is a 45-year-old woman who has been referred by a psychotherapist for treatment. The therapist has discussed the case with the practitioner, warning her that this woman has just suffered a great family tragedy and is very fragile. The therapist has recommended acupuncture as an adjunctive treatment since the patient suffers from a lot of physical, as well as emotional agitation. The patient goes from being depressed to laughing wildly to weeping uncontrollably.

The patient is so agitated that the practitioner is not able to take a pulse reading.

1. Differentiation of signs and symptoms:

2. Determination of the presence or absence of exogenous pathogenic factors:

3. Determination of whether the disturbance is of the Zang–Fu or the meridians:

4. Eight Guiding Criteria evaluation of the clinical data:

5. Establishment of a working diagnosis:

6. Determination of the treatment principle:

7. Determination of the treatment strategy:

8. Selection of methods:

9. Selection of points (Resource: to self-check, see *Essentials* pp. 65–6, *The Web* pp. 212–16.)

* Next steps:

SUMMARY

You may have noticed in working through the clinical cases that in doing one or a few steps it was not possible to gain a clear picture of the presenting clinical problems or perceive the patterns of disharmony behind the myriad signs and symptoms. However, as you proceeded to using steps 4 and 5, the picture became clearer and a working diagnosis was arrived at which was more rooted.

In utilizing this step-by-step problem-solving approach and in organizing clinical data in this way, we develop useful and effective diagnostic 'habits' that enable us to internalize what we have learned about the syndromes of the Zang–Fu, meridian symptomalogies, etc. It also aids in categorizing clinical data in a clear fashion, and leads to a logical choice of treatment strategy and points based on a consistent diagnostic process. In this way, treatment planning is no longer a somewhat haphazard or 'intuited' process, nor is it the unthinking application of memorized treatments from a book. This process is very useful in learning the various syndromes and symptomatologies of Chinese pathology, and insures a level of consistency in the practitioner's approach. Finally, it in no way detracts from the style, tone and inclinations of the practitioner, but merely serves as a useful guide to rational treatment planning and follow-up.

The ultimate goal of this book has been to initiate a series of textbooks for the teaching and learning of traditional oriental principles, concepts and practices for Westerners, and in this, I hope it serves as a beginning.

While this textbook is directed to learning integration of traditional acupuncture principles for energetic western students and practitioners, there is a much more central issue, namely the reformulation of acupuncture energetics as a mindbody therapy at the centre of an emerging paradigm of health maintenance and well-being.

REFERENCES

1. Ted J. Kaptchuk, O.M.D., *The Web that has no Weaver: Understanding Chinese Medicine*, New York, Congdon & Weed, 1983, p.179.
2. Manfred Porkert, *The Essentials of Chinese Diagnostics*, Acta Medicinae Sinensis Chinese Medicine Publications, Ltd, Zurich, 1983, p.15.
3. Cf. Mark D. Seem, *The Journal of Traditional Acupuncture*, Vol. 2, 1982.
4. See Chapter 5 for a detailed exploration of organization of this data.

BIBLIOGRAPHY

Austin, Mary, *Acupuncture Therapy*. Turnstone Press, 1981.
Bensky, Dan and O'Connor, John, *Acupuncture: A Comprehensive Text*, Chicago: Eastland Press, 1981.
Cheung, C.S. and Lai, Yat-Ki, *Principles of Dialectical Differential Diagnosis and Treatment of Traditional Chinese Medicine*, San Francisco: Traditional Chinese Medical Publisher, 1980.
Essentials of Chinese Acupuncture, Beijing: Foreign Languages Press, 1980.
Kaptchuk, Ted J., *The Web that has no Weaver: Understanding Chinese Medicine*, New York: Congdon & Weed, 1982.
Low, Royston, *The Secondary Vessels of Acupuncture*, New York and Wellingborough: Thorsons Publishers, 1983.
Porkert, Manfred, *The Essentials of Chinese Diagnostics*, Zurich: Acta Medicinae Sinensis Chinese Medicine Publications Ltd, 1983.

APPENDIX

Answer Key to Clinical Cases.
1. Mary Jones: Invasion of the Lung by Pathogenic Wind.
2. Joseph Rollo: Damp Heat in the Gall-Bladder.
3. Jim Sanchez: Cold Damp in the Large Intestine or Damp Distressing the Spleen.
4. Susan Cohen: Excess Heat of the Small Intestines or, Heart Fire moving by Meridian to the Small Intestines.
5. Adrienne Jones: Retention of Damp Phlegm in the Lungs.
6. Sam Chong: Obstruction of Qi of the Small Intestine.
7. Karen Reinhardt: Damp Heat in the Bladder.
8. Susan Allman: Deficient Cold in the Stomach or Deficient Spleen Yang.
9. Thomas Callahan: Stagnation of Cold in the Liver Channel.
10. Jimmy Nakasawa: Cold in the Bladder.
11. Richard Spatz: Deficient Cold of the Small Intestine, or Deficient Spleen Qi.
12. Adrienne Jones: Retention of Phlegm Heat in the Lungs.
13. Ruth Feinberg: Hyperactivity of Fire of the Heart.
14. Regina Lim: Exhausted Fluid of the Large Intestine.
15. Rita Haaz: Depression of the Qi of the Liver.
16. Stuart Richardson: Weakness of the Qi of the Heart — Yang Xu.
17. Rick Lyman: Stirring of the Wind of the Liver by Heat.
18. Sally Wright: Stomach Fire Blazing.
19. Tony Sims: Insufficiency of Yang of the Kidney.
20. Nigel Thomas: Damp Heat Invading the Large Intestine or Damp Heat Dysentery.

21. Peter Carmichael: Invasion of Spleen by Cold Damp.
22. Stuart Richardson (see also case 16): Weakness of the Qi of the Heart — Exhausted Yang.
23. Roslyn O'Reilly: Insufficiency of Yin of the Kidney.
24. Lionel Harvey: Congealed Blood in the Stomach.
25. Ralph Costello: Insufficiency of Yin of the Lungs.
26. Sam Jarvis: Intestinal Abscess — Appendicitis.
27. Nancy Sung: Deficient Qi of the Large Intestine.
28. Samuel Goldberg: Flare-up of the Fire of the Liver.
29. Jose Yamamoto: Stagnant Qi of the Small Intestine or, Cold Obstructing the Liver Meridian.
30. Siva Saraswati: Deficient Stomach Yin.
31. Samson White: Stagnation of Blood of the Heart.
32. Maria MacDonald: Weakness of Qi of the Spleen.
33. Tomoko Kanai: Insufficiency of the Blood of the Liver.
34. Ramona Santamaria: Insufficiency of Yin of the Heart.
35. Calhoun Alexander: Weakness of the Qi of the Kidney.
36. Rose Smith: Derangement of the Mind (a Heart syndrome).

INDEX